"Clever, vali
all at
— Tina Payne Bryson
co-au

The Untold Story!

EMMA AND THE E CLUB

An Epic Episode About Eliminating Enuresis and Encopresis

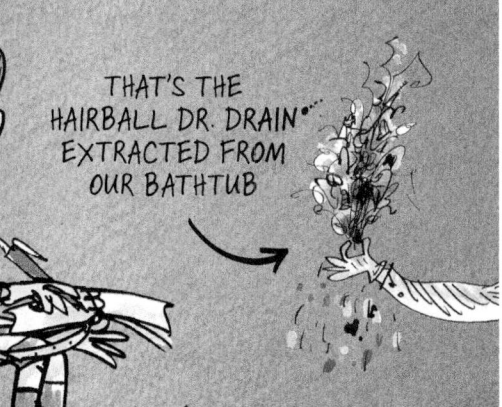

THIS IS ME, EMMA

THAT'S THE HAIRBALL DR. DRAIN EXTRACTED FROM OUR BATHTUB

BY SUZANNE SCHLOSBERG with Steve Hodges, M.D.
Illustrated by Mark Beech

> **Disclaimer**
> The information contained in this book is intended to supplement, not substitute for, the expertise and judgment of your physician or other health-care professional.

Emma and The E Club

Text Copyright © 2022 Suzanne Schlosberg with Steve J. Hodges

Illustration Copyright © 2022 Mark Beech

Book design: DyanRothDesign.com

ALL RIGHTS RESERVED. No part of this book may be reproduced or transmitted in any form by any means, electronic or mechanical, including photocopying and recording, or by any information storage and retrieval system, except as may be expressly permitted by the publisher. Requests for permission should be sent to permissions@oreganpress.com.

O'Regan Press

Library of Congress Cataloging-in-Publication Data is available on file.

979-8-9866795-0-1

This book is dedicated to Eden, whose
brave video about her encopresis treatment
inspired the character of Emma

WHAT KIDS ARE SAYING ABOUT EMMA AND THE E CLUB

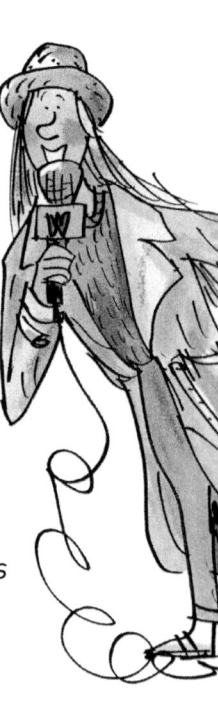

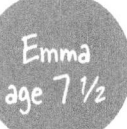
Emma age 7 ½

"This book is exceptional, a.k.a great! I'm ecstatic to learn about the E Club."

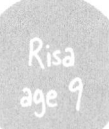
Risa age 9

"This book is one of the best books I've ever read. It made me feel so much better about my situation."

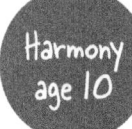
Harmony age 10

"I loved reading that accidents are not my fault. I hope this book will encourage other kids!"

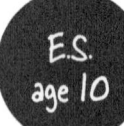
E.S. age 10

"This book explains everything I went through. Even though enemas might seem scary, they are actually one of your best friends and will make you feel 100 times better!"

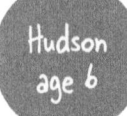
Hudson age 6

"This book will help other kids who feel nervous or anxious."

PRAISE FROM PARENTS

"My daughter devoured this book in one gulp! It's medicine for the soul of children with encopresis."
— David Spieser-Landis, Wilmington, North Carolina

"My twin boys thought Dr. Pooper was hilarious and were both really engaged."
— Vicky C., Tucson, Arizona

"My daughter enjoyed the whole storyline and got cross when I stopped reading."
— Claire H., Perth, Australia

"My son related to Emma and talked to her throughout the story. I loved the book, too, especially the E list and definitions."
— Rachel R., Pella, Iowa

"The book made my daughter feel more normal and less alone. She appreciated the humor, too."
— Jenni, Columbia, Missouri

"My 10-year-old said the book made her feel happy and less alone in her struggles. She loved the book and laughed out loud in many parts!"
— Meadow S., Petaluma, California

PRAISE FROM HEALTH PROFESSIONALS

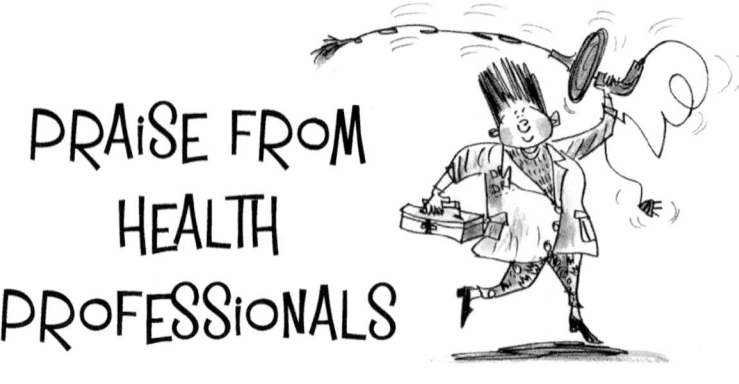

"A beautifully compassionate book, for both children and parents. The light-hearted tone makes a difficult topic easier to discuss."
— Laura Froyen, Ph.D. Respectful Parenting Educator, The Balanced Parent Podcast, Madison, Wisconsin

"Absolutely adorable! Perfect for my school-aged patients with pee and poop accidents. I love the addition of games at the end."
— Austin Grayce Hester, M.D. Pediatric Urologist, MUSC Shawn Jenkins Children's Hospital, Charleston, South Carolina

"A middle-grade novel that makes kids with encopresis and enuresis feel supported and understood. I'm thrilled!"
— Amanda Arthur-Stanley, Ph.D., Child Psychologist, Denver, Colorado

"Unique and entertaining! Addresses a common medical problem in a way that's easy to understand."
— Nadia Day, M.D., Pediatrician, Pediatric Associates, Phoenix, Arizona

"Explains a sensitive topic in a developmentally friendly, educational way."
— Cheyenne Hendrix, Certified Child Life Specialist Brenner Children's Hospital, Winston-Salem, North Carolina

"This book is sure to help kids with enuresis regain lost confidence."
— Dawn Sandalcidi, P.T., Pediatric Pelvic Floor Physical Therapist, Physical Therapy Specialists, Centennial, Colorado

Acknowledgments

First and foremost, I owe thanks to editor John Fox of Bookfox, who insisted I rework the entire manuscript and who was totally right about everything. Thank you for pushing me do all that extra work!

I am also thankful to my son Ian Spencer, who took the time to read the manuscript carefully and whose critiques were spot on. Ian also vetted the illustrations and made sure they passed the chuckle test.

Psychologist Amanda Arthur-Stanley offered valuable insights and sparked numerous ideas for the story.

Illustrator Mark Beech was a gem to work with and a real find! As always, our graphic designer, Dyan R. Roth, has shown herself to be as patient and meticulous as she is talented.

Proofreaders Emily Sandack and Judy Schlosberg found oodles of mistakes. Nice work!

Finally, I am grateful to the parents in our private Facebook support group who served as test readers for this book and especially to their children, whose comments greatly influenced the manuscript. I would like to credit the following kids as contributing editors:

- Eden S.
- Emma H.
- Silas R.
- Jordyn L.
- Phillip C.
- Hudson C.

— Suzanne Schlosberg

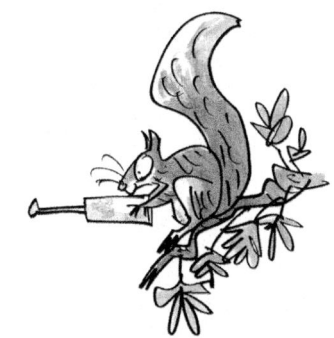

CONTENTS

Emma and the E Club

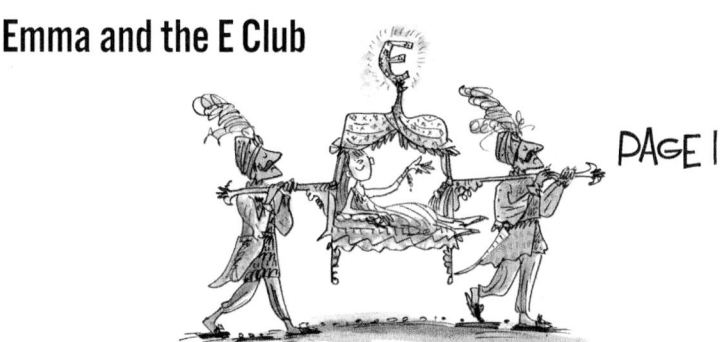

PAGE I

Emma's E Words

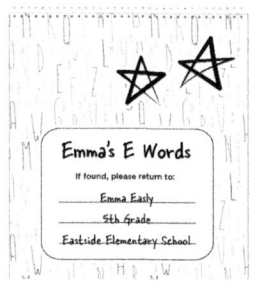

PAGE III

Emma's Word Games

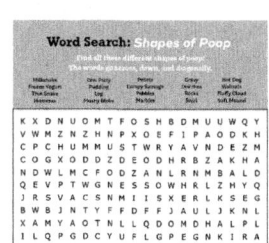

PAGE 125

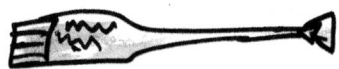

CHAPTER 1

Hi, I'm Emma Easly, and I'm the chief **executive** of the E Club. That means I'm in charge. I'm ten and a half and in fifth grade, and the club was **entirely** my idea.

I **expect** you want to know what the E stands for.

Well, for one thing, E stands for **enuresis**. That's the official name for pee accidents, **either** overnight or during the day.

E also stands for **encopresis**. That means you have poop accidents.

The E club is for kids who have enuresis or encopresis. Or both, like me.

I've had enuresis and encopresis most of my life, but until this year, I didn't **even** know accidents *had* official names. I just thought accidents were, you know, *accidents*—**embarrassing episodes** that pretty much only happened to me.

But I was in **error**! It turns out lots of kids, **everywhere** in the world, have enuresis and encopresis. It's just that no one talks about it.

Well, **except** me, **evidently**! I'm an **extrovert**, as you can tell. I've always been outgoing, and I like to think out loud.

You've probably noticed I **elect** to use words that start with E. That's because 1.) my first and last names both start with E and 2.) I **enjoy** playing with words. In fact, I

excel at it. That's not an **exaggeration**!

I'm **endlessly entertained** by word searches, crossword puzzles, and word scrambles. For **example**, I found forty-six words using the letters in "encopresis."
In this game, you can use any of the letters in any order. (Try it!)

Some words I found **easily**, like these:

CORN

NICE

OPEN

Other words took more **effort**:

NOISE

CRISP

SCORE

I even found an **eight-letter** word:

PRINCESS

Excellent, *eh?* You can check my work!

When I grow up, I plan to be **employed** as an **essayist**. That's a writer who **expresses** opinions.

I have a *lot* of opinions.

For example, in my **estimation**, a.k.a. my opinion, 1.) red licorice is superior to black licorice (which is barely even **edible**), and 2.) my mom **exaggerates** how much she **exercises**.

In case you weren't sure, a.k.a. stands for "also known as." My aunt, Jennifer, says "a.k.a." all the time, and I've started **emulating** her, a.k.a. being a copycat.

For example, yesterday Aunt Jennifer said, "Emma, my haircut is a catastrophe, a.k.a. a total disaster, a.k.a. I look like an **English** sheepdog."

She did. Her bangs **extended** into her **eyes**,

like a mop. I agreed with her, but she didn't seem happy about it.

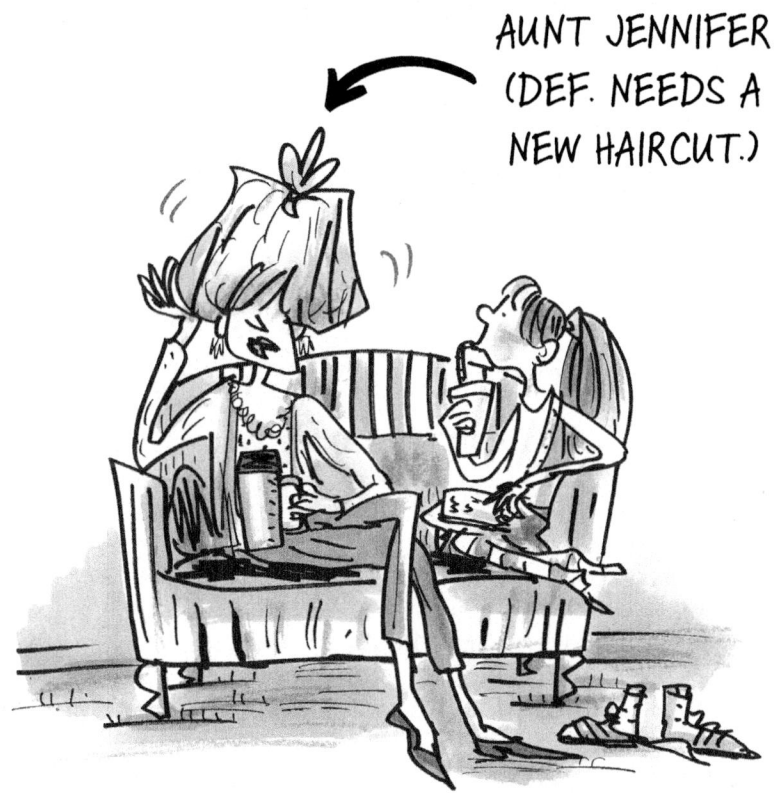

For fun, I collect words that start with E. In fact, I have an **enormous** list of E words—1,038 as of today.

Whenever I **encounter** an **E** word, I **enter** it into my notebook. I've clipped the notebook to a shoulder strap, so I **essentially** wear it, like a purse. I keep my **E** list handy at all times, except during recess, P.E., and soccer. I doodle in my notebook and draw a ★ next to words I didn't know before.

One new word on my list is **enema**. An enema is a treatment that helps you poop. My doctor told me about it. You squeeze medicine up your bottom through a small tube.

You're probably thinking: *Ewwww!*

That's **exactly** what I thought. To be honest, **enemas** do feel strange at first, but they don't hurt. I was surprised about that.

There's one kid in the E club, Lucas, who hasn't had an enema. So far, Lucas has been **emphatic**.

"No way," he told me. "*Not* happening."

"Never," he added. "In case I didn't make myself clear."

"Oh, you *did*," I replied. "One hundred percent."

CHAPTER 2

Want to know how the E Club got **established**?

One day I was at Food 4 Even Less supermarket with my mom. We had an **extensive** shopping list, including fruit, vegetables, beans, pasta, laundry soap, toothpaste, and enemas, **etc**. I hid the enema boxes under a bunch of bananas.

En route to the pasta aisle, we **encountered** our neighbor Charlotte and her mom. Charlotte is nine and a half and in fourth grade. She has super long hair and usually wears a pink felt hat with a roll-up brim. Once, I tried on her hat, but it bumped up against my ponytail. Let's just say it was not a good look.

At school Charlotte is **eminent**, a.k.a. famous, because she won the Invention Convention. Charlotte invented the Smart Scraper, a washable glove with an **edge** attached to one finger. The glove **enables** you to scrape the **entire** inside of a jar without getting peanut butter or jelly on your knuckles.

Genius, eh? But Charlotte isn't **egotistical** at all. She doesn't brag.

I looked at Charlotte's shopping cart and **eyed** three boxes of enemas—the same enemas I was using!

At the **exact** same time, while our moms were chit-chatting, probably about how much they've been "**exercising**" lately, Charlotte noticed the enemas in our basket, buried under the bananas.

We **exchanged expressions** like, "Wow, you *too?*" Then we exchanged smiles. In that moment, I knew we'd be great friends.

Feeling **emboldened**, a.k.a. daring, I whispered to Charlotte, "I used to think I was the only kid who had to use enemas. I have enuresis and encopresis."

Charlotte whispered back, "Really? I have enuresis, too. I didn't know other kids did enemas."

Just then, I had an **epiphany**, a.k.a. a sudden inspiration.

"We should start a club!" I said to Charlotte.

Charlotte **endorsed** the idea.

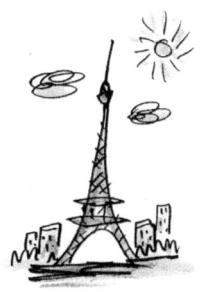

CHAPTER 3

The E Club meets in my treehouse. My dad built it last summer, when he **entered** into a contest with my uncle over who could **erect** the most **epic edifice**, a.k.a. building.

My dad thinks *he* won. My uncle thinks *he* won. In my opinion, the two treehouses are **equivalent**—about **equal**. I mean, they're not the **Eiffel** Tower or the **Empire** State Building, but for treehouses, they're pretty **elaborate**, a.k.a. fancy.

For example, my treehouse has a doorway curtain made entirely of beads. **Elegant**, eh? The curtain wasn't **expensive** at all. My mom bought it on **Etsy**.

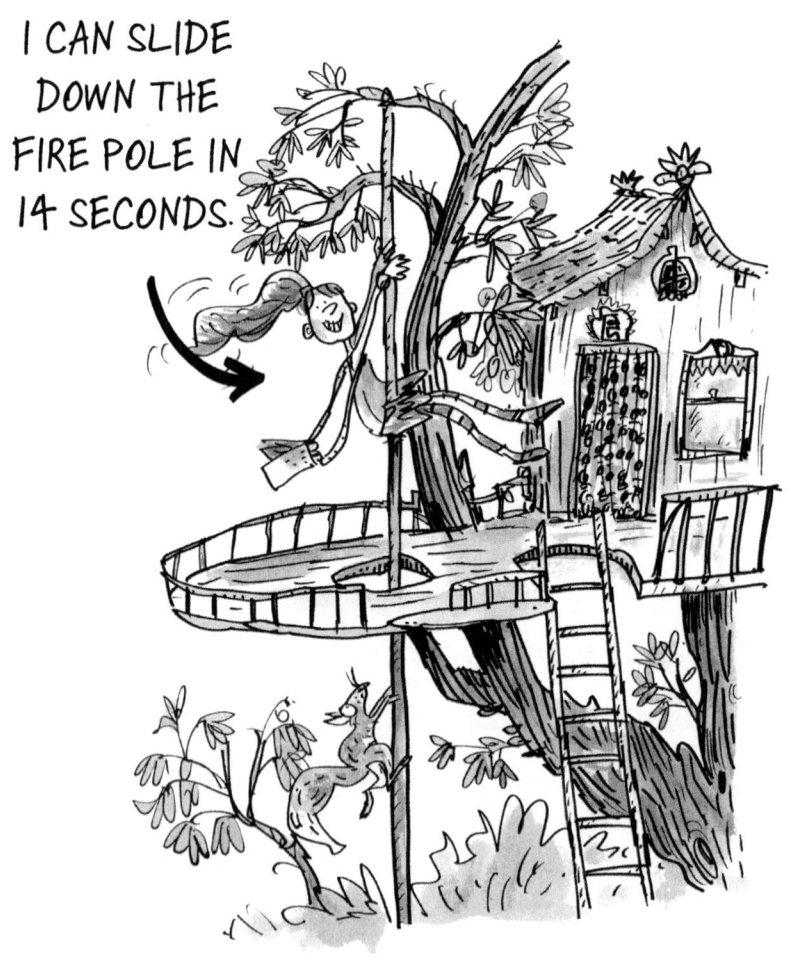

My treehouse is also **equipped** with a balcony and a fire pole. I slide down the pole if I need to get to the bathroom **expeditiously**, a.k.a. super fast.

I can make it from the treehouse to my bathroom in fourteen seconds flat. Jasmine, my next-door neighbor and best friend, timed me using my potty watch. My potty watch looks exactly like a regular watch, but it vibrates **every** two hours to remind me to pee.

Jasmine doesn't know about my enuresis and encopresis. I told her I wear a watch because I like knowing the exact time, which is true. She doesn't need to know the other reason.

Nobody knows about that except my parents, my doctor, and the other kids in the E Club, Charlotte and Lucas. Maybe you'll want to join! Any kid with encopresis or enuresis is invited. All ages are **eligible**.

We're **eager** to **expand** our club because we need help!

Our mission is to **eradicate**, a.k.a. wipe out, encopresis and enuresis. We **envision** a world where kids never have accidents at school or at birthday parties or anywhere else. A world where all kids can go on sleepovers without pull-ups or without worrying.

Are you wondering how the E Club is going to accomplish that? Well, we have a plan.

First, we're going to make an **exposé**. *Exposé* is a French word that's pronounced "EX-po-zay," and it means a shocking report that uncovers the truth.

For example, my mom and I once watched an exposé on TV called "Confessions of a Guilty Grandma." It was about a grandma nicknamed The Purse Lady who sold fake "designer" handbags—cheap, flimsy copycats. The police found 3,000 purses hidden in her garage!

"My purse broke apart the first week!" one of the Purse Lady's customers told the host of the show. "I got scammed."

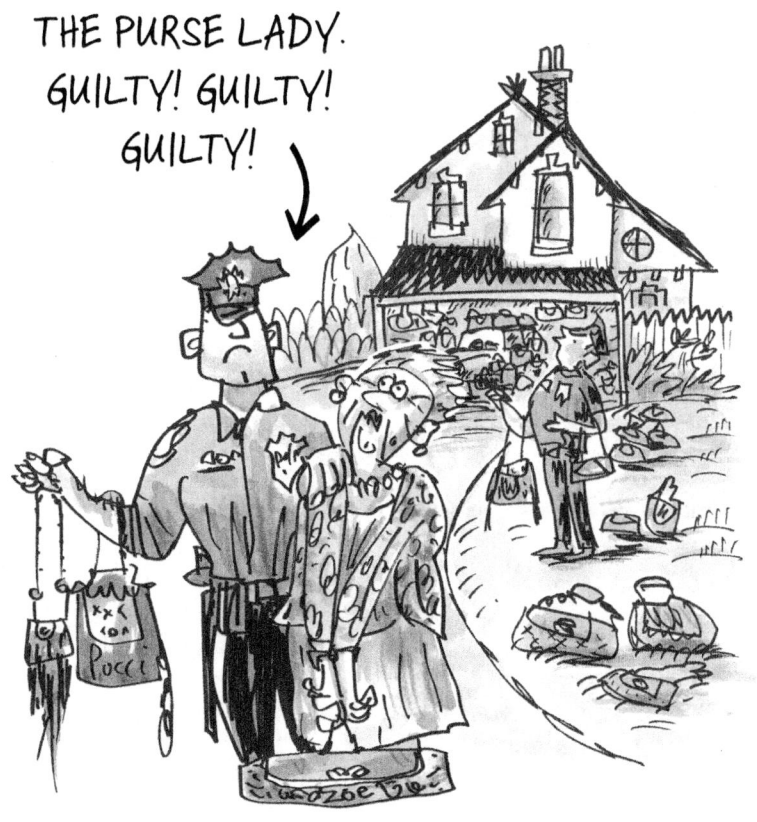

The Purse Lady spent her **earnings** on **extravagant** trips to **exotic** locations, like luxury cruises to tropical islands. Now she's in jail.

I was shocked to find out that a seventy-year-old with six grandchildren and a Labradoodle would trick people like that. *My* grandma never would. Definitely not!

Before I watched The Purse Lady show, I didn't even know copycat handbags **existed**. Now I know. Now **everyone** knows. Now, people will be more careful and buy their purses from actual retail **establishments**, a.k.a. real stores, not from some grandma who seems nice.

The E Club's exposé will be dramatic and **exciting**, like "Confessions of a Guilty Grandma." But our goal is to help kids rather than purse customers—a more important **endeavor**, in my opinion. We're going to reveal the truth about enuresis and encopresis: that accidents are never a kid's fault.

I have something **else** to tell you, a secret between Charlotte and me. We have another mission: to convince Lucas to try an enema.

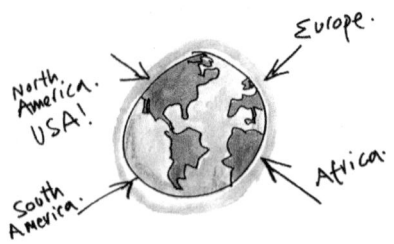

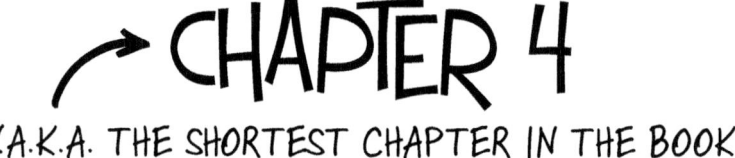

(A.K.A. THE SHORTEST CHAPTER IN THE BOOK)

When I was in third grade, I had a poop accident during math.

I didn't even feel the accident. Not one bit. My frenemy, Sammy, announced to the class, "Ewwww, Emma smells."

I felt my face get hot and turn bright red. Ms. Silverberg sent me to the school nurse.

The entire **experience** was **excruciating**—worse than painful.

I wanted to **escape** from school. From **Earth**, actually. In fact, I wanted to **exile**, a.k.a. banish, myself to Jupiter. Or **Europa**, one of Jupiter's icy moons.

I wished I didn't **exist**.

That's all I plan to say about this particular **event**. **Ever**.

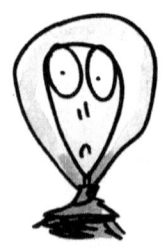

CHAPTER 5

In my estimation, if you're going to start a club, you need 1.) a mission and 2.) **enough** members.

The E Club had a mission. But let's face it: a club with two people isn't really a club. It's just two people hanging out.

"We need a third person," I said to Charlotte one afternoon, when we were up in the treehouse brainstorming ideas for our exposé.

Charlotte **echoed** my sentiment, a.k.a. totally agreed.

"But how will we find another member?" I said. "It's not like we're going to post a sign at school that says: *Do you have enuresis or encopresis? Join the E Club! Ask Emma and Charlotte about it!*"

But the very next day, we lucked out. I spotted a possible **enlistee**, a.k.a. new member, right on the school playground.

A bunch of us were playing zombie tag at lunch recess when I got tagged by Lucas. Lucas is in fifth grade, too, but this year he's not in my class. Lucas plays flag football and basketball and wears shorts every day, even when it's snowing. He's an **exceptionally** fast runner, and he always wins zombie tag. I'm not sure how Lucas can see anyone to tag, since his hair flops down over his eyes, sort of like Aunt Jennifer's. At least Lucas doesn't look like a sheepdog.

Anyway, right after Lucas tagged me, I

happened to glance at his wrist. I couldn't believe it: Lucas was wearing the same watch as me!

I had a **eureka** moment, a.k.a. a sudden realization: Maybe Lucas has enuresis or encopresis! I mean, that's the main reason kids wear vibrating potty watches.

Of course, I couldn't be sure. I didn't want to **embarrass** Lucas. Or myself.

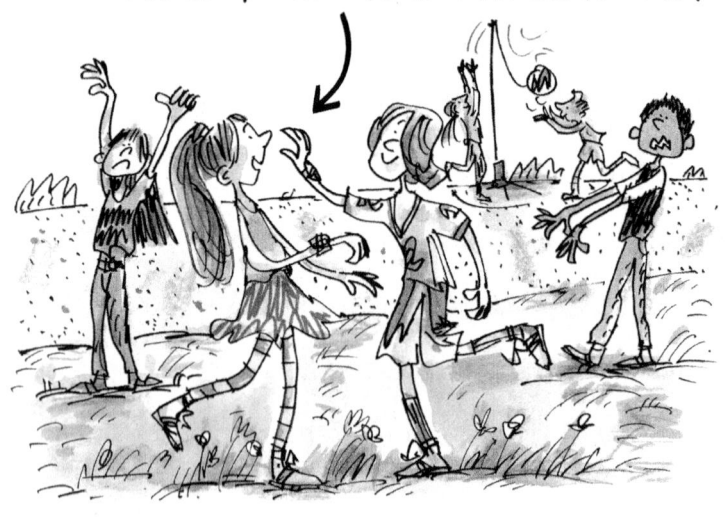

MY EUREKA MOMENT: LUCAS WAS WEARING THE SAME WATCH AS ME!

After zombie tag, I casually followed Lucas over to the tetherball pole. I whispered **extra** softly, so nobody could **eavesdrop**, "Hey, Lucas. I have the same watch. I wear it because I have enuresis and encopresis. Well, I used to, anyway."

Lucas seemed stunned I would share such private information. Honestly, I was kind of surprised myself. But the words just **emanated** from my mouth. I guess I was super determined to **enlist** a third member in the E Club.

Besides, I like Lucas. In fourth grade, we were table partners in science. He always shared the work **equitably**, a.k.a. fairly—unlike Olive and Violet, our other table partners, who **expected** Lucas and me to **exert** all the effort.

I felt I could **entrust** Lucas with my secret.

Feeling brave, I whispered, "Hey, do you ever have accidents?"

Lucas was **evasive**—a.k.a. he wouldn't answer.

"Well, in case you do," I said, "you could join the E Club. It's a club I started with Charlotte."

Lucas looked at me like I was an **extraterrestrial**. Like he had never heard an idea so strange.

"The E stands for *enuresis* and *encopresis*," I whispered. "It could also stand for *enema*. Have you ever had one?"

That was when Lucas sprinted off, faster than I had ever seen him run.

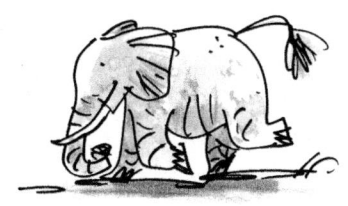

CHAPTER 6

For many years, my accidents were an **enigma** to me, a.k.a. a big mystery. I had no **earthly** idea why I kept peeing and pooping in my pants. It made no sense.

I mean, I *know* how to use the toilet. I learned when I was two!

By third grade, I could chop an onion, flip an omelet, and peel an **eggplant**. I could wash and dry my laundry, too. By fourth grade, I was our soccer team's best goalie. Once, I blocked a shot with **eight** seconds left in the game, **earning** our team a victory.

So, why couldn't I do something as simple as keep my pants dry?

My mom and dad never **explicitly** blamed me for my accidents. They never said, "Emma, stop wetting your bed." Of course not. They knew I didn't *want* to have accidents, and they tried to **empathize**.

Still, they seemed to feel I was responsible, at least to some **extent**. I saw their **eye-rolling** and heard their sighs.

My mom would say, "Emma, listen to your body! When you get the signal to pee or poop, go right to the toilet!"

"But my body isn't getting the signal!" I **exclaimed**. "I don't feel anything!"

My parents seemed **exasperated**, like I was purposely "waiting too long" and not "taking responsibility."

"Untrue!" I told my mom. "I take **exception** to that assumption."

In my estimation, 1.) no kid would ever poop or pee in their pants on purpose, and 2.) my mom was **egregiously**, a.k.a. terribly, uninformed.

My family tried **everything** to make my accidents stop.

My mom would wake me in the middle of the night to pee. That left both of us **exhausted**, but it didn't keep my sheets dry.

My dad suggested I stop drinking water in the **evenings**. That didn't help, either. It just made me thirsty.

Once, my grandma bribed me. She promised

to take me out for **éclairs**—fancy French pastries filled with cream and iced with chocolate—if I could go an entire week without an accident.

"You can do it, Emma!" she cheered. "I know you can!"

But I couldn't.

Every morning, I felt like a disappointment to my family and myself.

I would bolt out of bed, stuff my sheets in the washing machine, and try to **erase** the **episode** from my memory.

I'd say to Ernest, my **elephant** pillow pet, "Ernest, you know this isn't my fault, right?"

Ernest knew.

———

My parents and I expected my accidents to stop a long time ago. So did my first doctor. At my kindergarten checkup, she said **earnestly**, "Don't worry, Emma. You'll outgrow it."

She said the same thing at my **exams** in first grade, second grade, and third grade, too. She even said, "Don't worry," at my fourth-grade checkup.

But I *did* worry. Nothing had changed. How could I not worry?

No matter how much effort I **exerted**—no matter how hard I tried—dryness **eluded** me.

Every night I wet my bed. Most days, I had either a pee accident or a poop accident. Or both. Sometimes, I would **erupt** in tears.

One time, my mom said to my dad, "Maybe Emma's stressed out. Maybe something's bothering her, and that's why she's having accidents."

I **eavesdropped** on them from my bedroom. Then I **emerged** from the doorway and said, "No, Mom. You have it backwards. I'm not having accidents because I'm stressed. I'm stressed because I'm having accidents. If you had accidents, you'd be stressed, too."

Last spring, Jasmine invited me to a slumber party. I told her I had a previous **engagement** with my grandparents, but that was just an **excuse**.

The truth was, I was afraid of having an accident at Jasmine's house. Plus, I didn't want to risk my pull-ups being **exposed** for everyone to see.

Because of my encopresis and enuresis, I felt **excluded** from fun activities. I know that nobody was *actually* **excluding** me. I could have just hidden my pull-ups at sleepovers, like Charlotte did. But to be honest, my accidents were **eroding** my self-esteem. I was feeling down about myself.

I've never told that to anyone except Ernest. The E Club kids know, too.

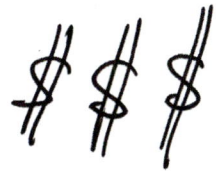

CHAPTER 7

Last winter, my mom broke her leg carrying an **extra-large** pizza box up our icy driveway, and she was stuck in bed for three weeks with her leg **elevated** on a pile of pillows.

During that time, she watched thirty-two episodes of *Unsolved Mysteries*, plus a series about famous prison **escapes** and an exposé about a mom who **embezzled**, a.k.a. stole, $100 million from the bank where she worked.

What I'm saying is, my mom is obsessed with

crime investigations.

She endlessly watches *Law & Order* reruns and Icelandic detective shows with subtitles. She listens to investigative podcasts while she **empties** the dishwasher—she's always wearing **earbuds**!

Whenever we visit the library, she **encourages** me to check out **Encyclopedia** Brown books. She's like, "Oh, Emma! I *adored* Encyclopedia Brown when I was your age. That series was my *favorite*."

Eh, it's OK. It's about a ten-year-old who solves crimes out of his garage "for twenty-five cents plus **expenses**." In my estimation, 1.) the clues are obvious and 2.) the cases are silly, **especially** "The Case of the Kidnapped Pigs."

Anyway, I've read loads of mysteries and watched **exposés** with my mom, so I know how to conduct an investigation.

For example, I know you "can't assume facts not in **evidence**"—a.k.a. you can't assume something is true unless you have proof.

I know you have to **evaluate** *all* the facts so you don't accuse people **erroneously**, a.k.a. falsely.

I know that mistaken ideas can become **entrenched**, a.k.a. stuck, in people's minds.

Here's what else I know: to most people, the cause of encopresis and enuresis is a mystery.

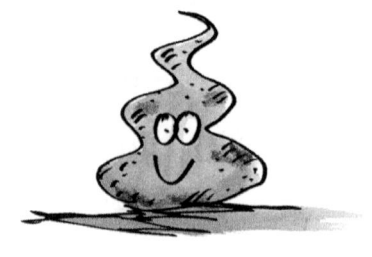

CHAPTER 8

You know how your entire life can change in a single day?

One Saturday in August, when I was seven, we moved to a new town and a new house, and I made a new best friend. All in one day!

That morning, our moving truck drove up while Jasmine was jumping rope on the sidewalk. She saw the movers unload my mom's **elliptical exercise** machine and sprinted across the grass toward me.

"Hey, my mom has one of those!" Jasmine exclaimed. "But she never uses it. She only *thinks* she does. She's in denial."

"Ha!" I said. "My mom uses our **electric easy** chair more than our elliptical, that's for sure. And FYI, I'm Emma. We moved because of my mom's job."

Later that day, Jasmine brought us homemade snickerdoodles, and I introduced her to Ernest. We've been best friends ever since.

That was an epic day.

At the start of fifth grade, I had another epic day: the day my mom and I met my new doctor.

His nickname is Dr. Pooper, and he's a urologist. A pee doctor. His entire job is to help kids **eliminate** enuresis and encopresis.

Dr. Pooper is 100% not like any other doctor I've met. For example, after he introduced himself, the first thing he said was, "Emma, how many different expressions do you know for pooping?"

"More than all the fifth-grade boys put together!" I replied.

"Is that so?" he said.

Dr. Pooper challenged me to a contest—a challenge I **eagerly** accepted. We took turns for quite a while.

"Bomb the bowl!" he said.

"Bake a loaf!" I said.

"Launch a torpedo!" he said.

"Lay a brick!" I said.

"Squeeze the cheese!" he said.

"Poke the turtle's head out!" I said.

"Download some software!" he said.

"Build a log cabin!" I said.

"Take the Browns to the Super Bowl!" he said.

My mom looked like she might **evaporate** from **embarrassment**. She had no idea my poop vocabulary was so extensive. She also didn't know the Browns are a football team in Cleveland.

Dr. Pooper seemed surprised I could keep up with him. Of course, he didn't know word games are my area of **expertise**, a.k.a. skill.

Soon he **escalated** our competition, talking even faster and switching to words that mean *poop*.

"Dung!" he said.

"Doo-doo!" I said.

"Dumplings!" he said.

"Droppings!" I said.

"Dingleberry!" he said.

"Doody!" I said.

"Snake!" he said.

"Cow patty!" I said.

"Chocolate hot dog!" he said.

"Excrement!" I said.
"Excreta!" he said.
That's when I **ended** the game.

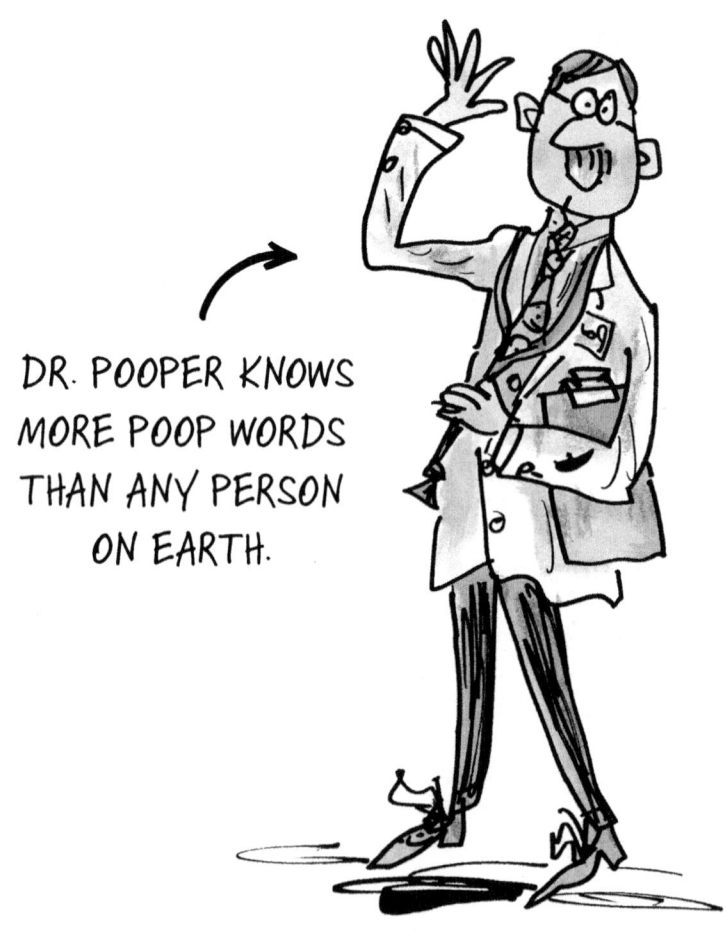

DR. POOPER KNOWS MORE POOP WORDS THAN ANY PERSON ON EARTH.

"Hold up a minute!" I interrupted, opening my E word notebook. "I need to write that last one down!"

I told Dr. Pooper about my E word collection. "A word **enthusiast**, *eh?*" he said. "You're quite the **erudite** one!"

I wrote down *erudite*, too. Dr. Pooper said it means "learned"—a.k.a. a person who has learned a lot. I guess I have!

During the **examination**, Dr. Pooper told me he'd had accidents in **elementary** school, too.

"A few kids were mean about it," he **empathized**. "I stopped using the school bathroom, but that only **exacerbated** my enuresis. Only made it worse."

I could relate. I did not like pooping in the school **environment**. Pooping sometime hurt, and I preferred the privacy of my bathroom at home.

The best part of my appointment was when Dr. Pooper said, "Emma, you know your accidents are *not* your fault, right?" He put a lot of **emphasis** on the word *not*.

"Excuse me?" I said. "Could you please repeat that?"

I wanted to **ensure** my mom had heard him.

"Well," he said, "when you have encopresis or enuresis, you can't feel the accidents coming. It's like a storm is headed your way but your warning system is on the fritz. You can't possibly get to the toilet in time."

Suddenly, I felt **exonerated**, a.k.a. proven innocent.

"Thank you for **enlightening** us," I said to Dr. Pooper.

I recognized the **expression** on my mom's face: It was like that *"Hmmm... interesting"* face that TV detectives make when they discover evidence that sends the investigation in a whole new direction.

I could see my mom's attitude was **evolving**, a.k.a. gradually changing. Still, she didn't seem entirely convinced.

"I can feel when *I* need to use the toilet. Why can't Emma?" she asked Dr. Pooper.

"Because she has constipation," he said.

"What?" my mom exclaimed. "Emma **eats** healthier than I do, and she plays soccer! She can't be constipated. Impossible!"

"Not just possible, Mrs. Easly," Dr. Pooper said, "but factual!"

Dr. Pooper had evidence.

CHAPTER 9
(A.K.A. THE LONGEST CHAPTER IN THE BOOK)

Last year, the pipe in our bathtub clogged up. At first, the water took **eons**, a.k.a. forever, to drain. When the tub stopped up entirely, my dad called the plumber.

That afternoon, an enormous white van pulled into our driveway. It looked exactly like an ambulance, with a red cross **emblazoned** on the **exterior**. The van said: "The Drain Doctor—**Emergency** Care."

My dad opened the front door, and there stood the plumber, a short woman with spiky hair. She was wearing a white doctor's coat, and "Dr. Drain" was **embroidered** in red on the pocket.

In my estimation, 1.) Dr. Drain was even more **eccentric**, a.k.a. peculiar, than Dr. Pooper, and 2.) her **ensemble**, a.k.a. outfit, was actually pretty funny.

DR. DRAIN AND HER EXCRUCIATINGLY LOUD ELECTRIC DRAIN SNAKE.

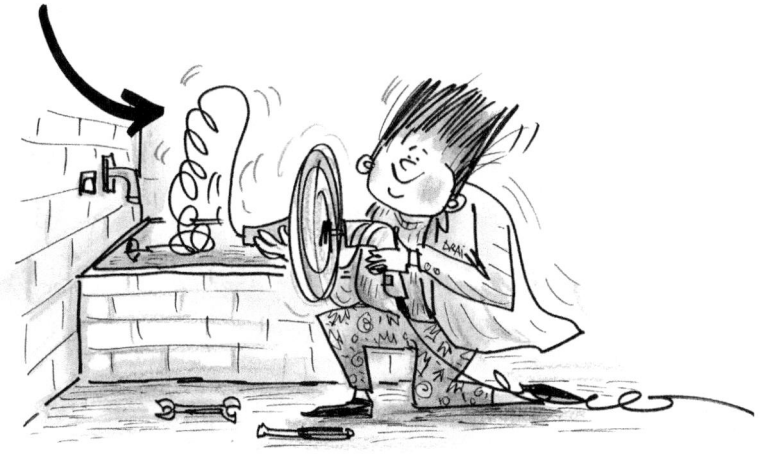

"Alrighty, I'm here to **examine** the patient!" she said, evidently referring to our bathtub.

Dr. Drain was holding a silver machine that looked like a tea kettle stuck to a power drill. She called it her "trusty electric drain snake."

I **escorted** Dr. Drain to the bathroom, where she plugged her **equipment** into the wall. Then she pulled a long, coiled metal cable out of the machine. That was the snake, I figured.

Dr. Drain flipped a switch, and—wowzers!!! The electric drain snake **elicited** an **earsplitting** noise, even louder than our Ninja Mega Jet II, the blender my mom uses to make "power smoothies" after she "exercises."

Then, Dr. Drain **expertly** inserted the snake into the bathtub pipe until it wouldn't go in any further.

"We have met the blockage!" she announced.

A few seconds later, she **extracted** a massive, **entangled** wad of hair from the pipe, and then **extricated**, a.k.a. carefully removed, the hairball from the snake's coils.

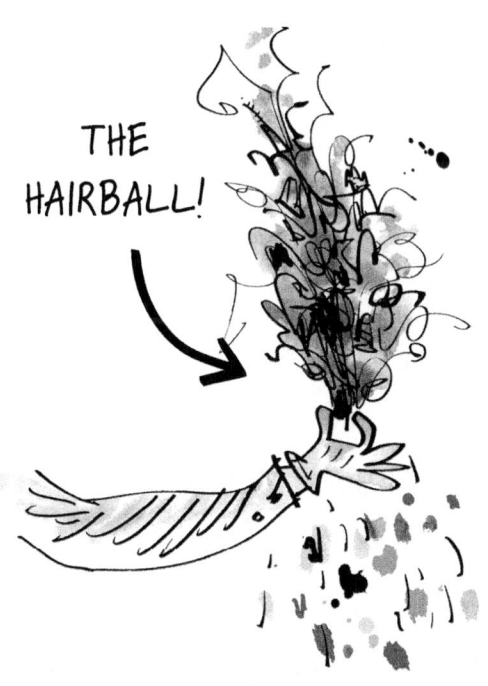

"No wonder your drain went kaput!" Dr. Drain said. "Patient never had a chance—not with a colossal clog like that. All healed now!"

If you're wondering what all this has to do with enuresis and encopresis, I'll tell you: What happened to our bathtub drain is what happened to me.

A pipe in my belly—a pipe called the rectum—got clogged. With poop.

"You're all stopped up," Dr. Pooper told me.

———

To prove I had constipation, Dr. Pooper **exhibited** my x-ray on a light board.

An x-ray is a picture of the inside of your body, only the picture is taken **externally**, a.k.a. on the outside. The x-ray machine sends waves of **energy**, called **electromagnetic** waves, through your skin.

My mom had an x-ray after her accident with the pizza box. You could see that she had broken her leg in two places.

On my x-ray, Dr. Pooper pointed to the rectum, the **end** of the colon.

"Emma, have you ever been to Chicago?" he asked. "The Windy City?"

"Nope," I said. "Why do you ask?"

"Because your rectum looks like the **Eisenhower Expressway** at rush hour! **Ensnarled** with traffic. All backed up! That highway's like a parking lot! Nothing moves!"

Dr. Pooper **explained** that your rectum isn't designed to hold loads of poop, just one day's worth.

"It's about the size of a toilet paper roll, not the giant handbag my wife hauls around," Dr. Pooper said. "I have no idea what she keeps in there!"

I hoped that Dr. Pooper's wife hadn't been

tricked into buying a fake designer handbag, like the Purse Lady's customers had.

"Every single day, your body cranks out fresh poop," Dr. Pooper continued, "so every day you've got to fully **evacuate**. It's **essential** to **expel** the entire load. I mean, turn on that **excavator** and dig!"

He turned to my mom and said, "Emma's only squeezing half the cheese! Downloading half the software!"

My mom looked 100% **embarrassed**. But Dr. Pooper was right.

"Sometimes I can only **eke** out a few chunks," I told him. "It feels like there's more inside, but it won't come out. Like it's stuck. Like I'm a clogged toilet. Like I'm trying to poop out cement."

Dr. Pooper pointed out that unlike a toilet

paper roll or bathtub pipe, your rectum is stretchy. So, when **excess** poop piles up, your rectum **expands**.

"Like an overstuffed **enchilada**!" he said.

Dr. Pooper motioned toward a poster on his wall **entitled**: YOU'RE GETTING ON MY NERVES (WELL, NOT YOU *PERSONALLY*).

He identified the bladder, the organ that holds your pee.

"Now, see how your rectum and your bladder are practically touching **each** other? Well, when your rectum becomes **enlarged**, it **encroaches** upon your bladder. Invades your bladder's space! Like my wife invades my space when she rolls over in bed. Squishes me!"

Dr. Pooper seemed to have as much **enthusiasm** for internal organs as Dr. Drain did for bathtub pipes.

"When your rectum presses against your bladder, that makes your bladder nerves go bonkers." Dr. Pooper said, making a batty face, with his **eyeballs** bulging, his nose wrinkled, and his tongue sticking out.

"When the nerves in your bladder are squished," he said, "your brain doesn't get the message that it's time to pee."

"The traffic light is broken! **Ergo**, you're totally out of the loop," he said.

"FYI," he added, "*ergo* means 'therefore.' In case you want to write it down."

I did.

Dr. Pooper got back on track. "Without bothering to warn you, your whacked-out bladder squeezes hard, and pee leaks out. It happens so fast that you can't make it stop. Like a sneeze."

That's exactly what I had **experienced**.

"FYI, that's why bribery never works, even though most parents try it," Dr. Pooper said. "That idea ought to be **expunged** from whatever parenting handbook it came from. **Erased**! Deleted!"

I gave my mom the **evil eye**—well, not exactly *evil*, but I did glare at her, the way she glares at me when I leave my room a mess. ("Emma, did an **earthquake** hit?" she'll say, frowning.)

Dr. Pooper continued, "Let's say you were home sick with a cold, Emma. Let's say your mom offered you two extra hours of screen time to go the whole day without sneezing. Would that work?"

"Definitely not," I said.

"Well, it's the same with enuresis," he said, shifting his glance from me to my mom. "A whacked-out bladder does not care about screen time or treats!"

I was grateful for this bit of **edification**, a.k.a. **education**.

"OK, but why am I having poop accidents? I asked. "And how come I can't even feel the poop coming out?"

This was when Dr. Pooper hopped onto the examination table and yanked off his shoe and his white tube sock. Then, he stuffed the sock with a wide roll of bandage wrapping.

"Emma, what would happen to my sock if I left it stuffed like this for months? Or years?"

"Um, it would stretch out and get saggy?" I guessed, shocked by this **exhibition**. "It would become less **elastic**?"

"Exactly!" Dr. Pooper said, putting his sock and shoe back on. "That's what happens to an overstuffed rectum. It becomes floppy. So, sometimes, a load drops right out."

He told me that when your rectum is saggy, you don't feel the urge to poop, so even more poop piles up.

"That makes your rectum stretch even more," Dr. Pooper said. "It's like an **endless** loop."

I was totally **engrossed** in, a.k.a. fascinated by, what Dr. Pooper had to say. I mean, this was **eye-popping, earth-shaking** information.

Suddenly, *everything* made sense—my stomachaches, my accidents, my entire life.

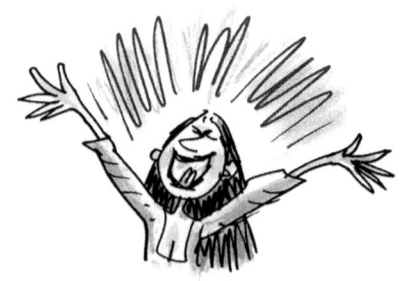

CHAPTER 10

The day after I asked about his potty watch, Lucas **evaded** my glance. Whenever I looked in his direction at recess, he would turn his head and go **elsewhere**.

In my estimation, this meant Lucas 1.) did have encopresis or enuresis (or both), and 2.) was afraid to try an enema.

I mean, I'm not a professional detective, but the clues were **evident**. Otherwise,

Lucas would have just said, "What in the world is an enema? I have no idea what you're talking about."

But I suspected Lucas knew *exactly* what I was talking about. He just wasn't interested in discussing it with me.

That was totally **excusable**. I mean, accidents are 100% the worst topic ever—if you're still having them.

Once your accidents stop, you're so **ecstatic**, a.k.a. thrilled, that you want all kids with enuresis or encopresis to know about enemas. At least I do.

Anyway, I didn't want to ruin Lucas's recess, so I joined the wall ball game while he played zombie tag.

After school in the treehouse, I told Charlotte about my conversation with Lucas. I worried that because of my big mouth, I had blown our chance to enlist Lucas in the E Club.

"I can't believe I asked Lucas if he'd ever had an enema!" I told Charlotte. "Who would ask a personal question like that?"

"Um, *you*, apparently," Charlotte said. "I bet in the entire history of the universe, nobody has ever said *enema* on a school playground."

"Lucas will probably never talk to me again," I said, regretting that I'd been such a blabbermouth.

"Maybe," Charlotte said. "But then again, maybe you've made him curious. If he's tired of having accidents, he might just be ready to try an enema."

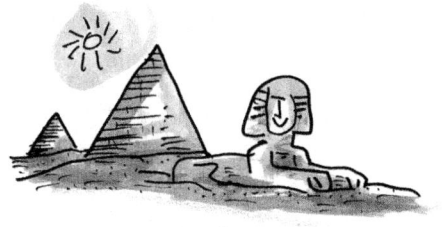

CHAPTER 11

Before I met Dr. Pooper, I had never heard of an enema. At first, I didn't even catch what he said. I thought he was not **enunciating**, a.k.a. speaking clearly.

"An **enemy**?" I said, confused.

"Nope!" he said. "An enema is *not* your enemy! When you have enuresis or encopresis, an enema is your friend."

Dr. Pooper handed me a squeeze bottle with a small tube attached.

"This here is an enema," he said. "The bottle is filled with medicine."

Then he showed me another type of enema, too: a squeezy tube with a larger end and a smaller end.

He explained that you insert the small end into your bum and squeeze the other end. While you wait for the medicine to start working, you **entertain** yourself in the bathroom.

"Watch a video or read a book or play with your **Etch** A Sketch!" he said.

He told me that after a few minutes, you feel an **extreme** urge to poop, a feeling you can't ignore. Then you sit on the toilet, and—*plop!* A load of poop is **expelled** from your bottom.

"Like a big ol' poop **extravaganza**!" Dr. Pooper said.

Even though enemas were new to me, Dr.

Pooper said they've existed for over 2,000 years.

"The ancient **Egyptians** used them!" he said. "That was before squeezy tubes were invented. You had to hollow out a gourd—a big squash. Or use a tube of bamboo attached to some goat skin."

I was glad I didn't live in ancient **Egypt**. I was thankful for squeezy tubes.

Dr. Pooper pointed to a giant book on his shelf titled *A History of Medicine,* where he apparently learned these **esoteric**, a.k.a. obscure, facts.

"You know what else?" he said. "Enemas were popular with the pharaohs, the **Egyptian** kings! Each pharaoh employed a Keeper of the Royal Rectum. His job was to prepare the pharaoh's enemas."

In my estimation, 1.) that did not sound like **enjoyable employment**, and 2.) Dr. Pooper owned some really boring books. I suggested he read *Harry Potter*.

Anyway, Dr. Pooper explained that enemas are an especially **effective** way to unclog your rectum.

"Some kids need an inhaler to help them breathe," Dr. Pooper said. "Some kids need tutoring to help them read. And some kids need enemas to help them poop. No one in life is **exempt** from needing a bit of assistance, Emma!"

He paused for a moment.

"And that includes me, FYI. For a while, I had to enlist my wife's help dressing for work, if you can believe that. I have an **eclectic** wardrobe—stripes, polka dots, plaid, paisley, you name it. Inside my closet, my wife taped pictures of all my ties and shirts and drew arrows showing which ones matched. **Eventually**, I figured it all out."

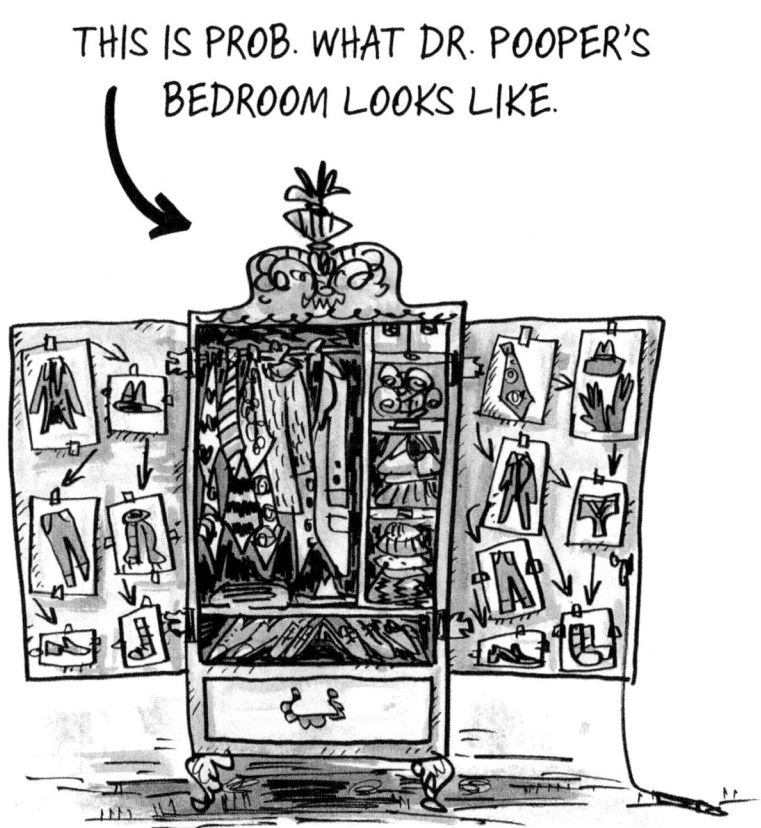

THIS IS PROB. WHAT DR. POOPER'S BEDROOM LOOKS LIKE.

Underneath his white coat, Dr. Pooper was wearing a blue and white striped shirt and a purple tie with tiny goldfish. I thought maybe his wife should still be helping him.

"Most of my patients use enemas," Dr. Pooper said. "It's no big deal."

My mom did not agree. She thought enemas sounded too "extreme."

That's when Dr. Pooper interjected. "Say, has your bathtub drain ever gotten clogged, Mrs. Easly?"

"Actually, last year," my mom replied.

"Did you think, *Oh, one day our wonderful drain will outgrow this clog*? Or did you call a plumber to snake out the hairball?"

I told Dr. Pooper all about Dr. Drain and her ambulance and her doctor's coat.

"**Enterprising** woman!" Dr. Pooper said. "Imaginative!"

Then he returned to the subject at hand.

"Bathtub drains don't unclog themselves," he said. "Neither do rectums."

"But isn't there an **easier** way?" my mom asked. "Couldn't Emma drink poop powder mixed with water? Wouldn't that make pooping easier for her and fix her constipation?"

"Indeed, for some children, poop powders and syrups do an **estimable** job," Dr. Pooper said. "They work A-OK. However, when a child has enuresis or encopresis, poop powder is often not **efficacious**."

Dr. Pooper nodded toward my notebook. "E-F-F-I-C-A-C-I-O-U-S—that's how you spell it, Emma," he said. "It means 'useful.' For lots of kids, poop powder just isn't useful."

"Why not?" my mom asked.

"Because the fresh, soft poop just oozes around the big, hard clog," Dr. Pooper replied.

I did not like the sound of "oozing."

"In fact," Dr. Pooper continued, "for children with encopresis, poop powder can make matters worse. You can end up with a big poopy mess!"

I *especially* did not like the sound of "big poopy mess." I'd had enough messes.

Dr. Pooper **enumerated**, a.k.a. counted off, the reasons my mom didn't need to worry.

"First off, enemas are gentle and safe," he said. "Second, the enema tip is a lot smaller than the giant bricks Emma's been squeezing out. Third, once Emma's accidents resolve, she won't need enemas anymore."

In my estimation, 1.) Dr. Pooper made a ton of sense, and 2.) my mom was overreacting.

As for me, I was **elated**, a.k.a. thrilled, because I knew that the sooner I started doing enemas, the sooner my accidents would stop.

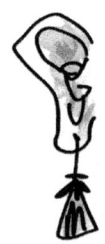

CHAPTER 12

For a few days, I didn't even try to talk to Lucas. I didn't look at him during recess. I stayed away from zombie tag and tetherball, Lucas's two favorite games.

So, I was 100% surprised one day when Lucas came up to me after wall ball and, when no one was around, whispered, "OK, fine."

"Fine?" I asked. "What's fine?"

"Sometimes I have accidents," Lucas said in

my **ear**. "Just at night."

I was **exultant**, a.k.a. overjoyed. I mean, obviously I wasn't happy Lucas had to **endure** accidents, but I was relieved to know he wasn't mad at me.

In his own way, Lucas was asking for help. Admirable, eh?

Now I just had to convince him to join the E Club.

I didn't want to scare him off by sounding too **excited**, so I acted casual and **easygoing**.

"Well, yeah, lots of kids have enuresis," I said. "You're lucky it only happens to you at night. At least you never had an accident in class, like I did."

My grandpa Julius's favorite **exhortation**, a.k.a. piece of advice, is, "Nothing's so bad that it couldn't be worse." Like, when my mom felt blue after her **escapade** with the pizza box, Grandpa

entreated her, a.k.a. urged her, to see the bright side of having a broken leg.

"Nothing's so bad that it couldn't be worse," Grandpa Julius said. "You could have broken both legs! Or your back!"

I thought Lucas might feel better if he realized some kids are even more unlucky.

The bell was about to ring, so I quickly invited Lucas to my treehouse the next day. I told him about the fire pole and the triple fudge brownies I was planning to bake for our meeting.

"Charlotte and I have a big **enterprise** we're working on," I said. "A big project. Will you help us?"

Lucas **equivocated**—a.k.a. he wouldn't commit.

"Um…" was all he said.

Just then, the bell rang. Lucas ran off without answering.

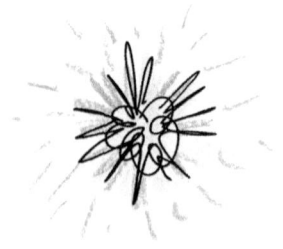

CHAPTER 13

To be honest, I wasn't 100% **enthusiastic** about **embarking** on the enema program Dr. Pooper had recommended. Even though he had **eased** my mind a lot, I still worried that inserting the tube would hurt.

My mom seemed to be more scared than I was, and she said I didn't have to do it.

"It's *entirely* your choice," she **emphasized**.

But the more I thought about it, the more I **embraced** the idea. I felt **empowered**, ready to take charge and do something daring.

I **envied** kids who wore underwear. Kids who went to sleepovers without worrying about accidents.

I was tired of pull-ups and wet sheets.

"*Enough* already!" I told Ernest one night.

My mom wanted to help me with the enema, but I **elected** to do it myself.

The first time I gave myself an enema, I was on edge, a.k.a. super nervous. My mom and I reviewed the instructions, and then she **exited** the bathroom.

Dr. Pooper had told me the tip slides in more easily if you use extra lubricant. "Use a big gob!" he'd said. "The size of the Death Star!"

He also said it helps if your pooping muscles are relaxed—if you **exhale** forcefully, like you're blowing out birthday candles.

My mom calls it "yoga breathing," even though she never does yoga.

Right before I inserted the enema, I said out loud, "I am brave. I am strong. I am Emma."

"You certainly are!" my mom replied, from outside the bathroom.

You know what? The enema was entirely **endurable**. I could totally deal with it.

About three minutes later, I got the signal—the "urge," my mom calls it—and a big load of poop was **ejected** from my bottom. It was **explosive**, if you really want to know. Like a volcanic **eruption**.

Afterward, I felt a million times better.

———

It only took me a few days to get used to enemas. Now, I'm an **expert**. I can "**enemize**"—a.k.a. give myself an enema—**effortlessly**.

FYI, I added *enemize* to my notebook, even

though I made up the word.

"Emma the **Enemizer**," I call myself.

"Emma the Enemizer **Extraordinaire**!" Dr. Pooper calls me.

Actually, he has lots of different titles for me. He tries them out when I visit his office.

"Well, if it isn't Her **Excellency**, the **Esteemed** Queen of the Royal Rectum!" he'll say.

HER EXCELLENCY, THE EXALTED EMPRESS OF THE ENEMA EMPIRE.

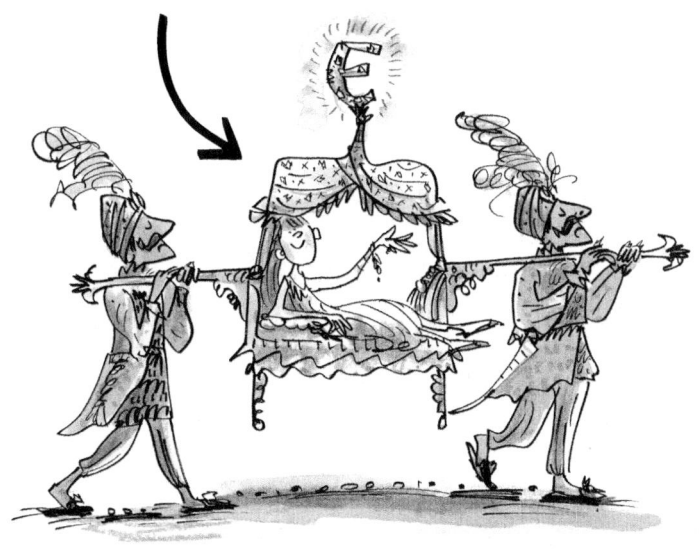

"Greetings, Emma the **Exalted Empress** of the Enema Empire! I'm **enchanted** to resume our acquaintance!"

Another time he called me "Emma of the Upper **Echelon**."

"*Echelon* means 'level,'" Dr. Pooper clarified. "You are top level, Emma! The very top!"

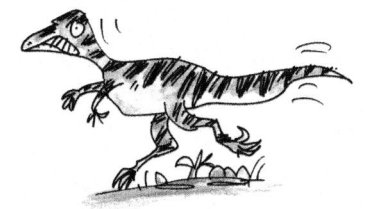

CHAPTER 14

I wasn't surprised when I heard Lucas climbing the treehouse ladder.

A day **earlier**, my mom had called Lucas's mom to **explain** the E Club. Lucas's mom told my mom that they had visited Dr. Pooper, too, but that Lucas **eschewed** the idea of enemas—a.k.a. he wanted nothing to do with them.

Lucas's mom hoped that joining the E Club might **encourage** Lucas to change his mind. But mostly she wanted Lucas to hang with other kids who'd had the same **experiences**.

In my estimation, 1.) Lucas's mom probably bribed him to come our meeting, and 2.) the bribe probably involved extra screen time.

None of that mattered. I was glad Lucas came.

"Is this where the triple fudge brownies are?" Lucas said, popping his head through the beaded doorway.

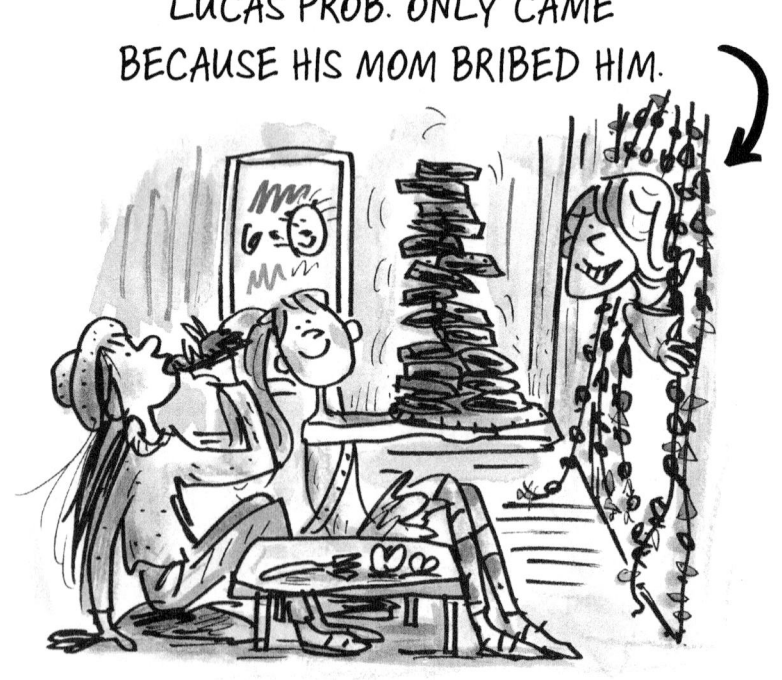
LUCAS PROB. ONLY CAME BECAUSE HIS MOM BRIBED HIM.

"You're in the right place!" I said, offering him the plate. "I actually made them quadruply fudgy."

Even though Lucas wasn't **enthused** about the meeting, he was **effusive**, a.k.a. complimentary, about my brownies.

"Not bad, Emma," he said. "Not bad at all."

I had an **eventful** meeting planned for us—we had lots to discuss.

First, I explained the exposé idea to Lucas. He had no clue what I was talking about. Evidently, his mom did not watch *Dateline* and *Cold Case Files*.

So, I **expounded** on my idea—a.k.a. I told him more about it.

"We're going to call it 'Constipation Investigation: The Untold Story!'" I said. "With an **exclamation** point, so it sounds exciting."

I explained that each episode would **expose** a "shocking truth" about encopresis or enuresis.

"For example," I said, "most people don't even know accidents are caused by constipation. They invent all kinds of **explanations**—explanations that are not logical or backed up by evidence."

"That's for sure," Charlotte said.

Charlotte's first-grade teacher had blamed Charlotte's accidents on her "refusal" to use the toilet at recess and had called Charlotte "disruptive" for asking to use the bathroom during class.

If you ask me, the expression *potty refusal* should go **extinct**. I'd like to **enact** a law against using it! I mean, you can't "refuse" to follow a signal that you're not even getting.

One doctor told Charlotte's mom, "Charlotte will stop having accidents when she's ready."

"Can you believe that?" Charlotte told Lucas

and me. "What kid isn't ready to stop having accidents?"

Another doctor said Charlotte was wetting her bed because she's a deep sleeper.

Actually, my first doctor had said that about me, too. Dr. Pooper said that theory is popular but **erroneous**.

"It doesn't matter if you can sleep through the roar of a jet **engine** or the screech of an **enraged** Tasmanian devil!" Dr. Pooper explained. "If your bladder is healthy and stable—if the nerves haven't gone haywire—you simply will not need to pee overnight."

He added, "Being a deep sleeper can't make your bladder go bananas!"

I wanted to **educate** the world about enuresis and encopresis. I wanted kids to get treatment instead of getting blamed or ignored.

"That's the untold story I want the E Club to tell!" I said. "My mom said she'll post our show on the internet, for maximum **exposure**—so everyone can watch!"

"No way!" Lucas exclaimed. "I don't want to be seen on the internet talking about accidents!"

"You don't have to be on camera," I replied. "You can be the person *holding* the camera. My mom said we can use her phone. No one will even know you were involved."

Charlotte, on the other hand, wanted to star in the show.

"Can I be the host?" she asked.

Charlotte 100% had my **endorsement**, a.k.a. my support. She has an **exuberant** personality—she's cheerful and **energetic**—and she speaks **eloquently**. She really gets people to listen.

When Charlotte demonstrated the Super

Scraper at the Invention Convention, she was highly **entertaining**. Everyone wanted to buy one of her gloves! Of course, they weren't for sale.

I'm more of a behind-the-scenes kind of person. I planned to be the show's script writer and video **editor**. That's the person who decides which parts to keep in the show and which parts are **expendable**, a.k.a. not needed.

I turned to Lucas. "I have a second job for you, Lucas. Will you choose the music?"

Lucas plays the electric guitar, and his band, The Rotten Apples, performed at our school variety show last year. He's super talented and can play everything from **Elvis** to **Eminem**.

"For dramatic **effect**, every exposé needs suspenseful music," I said. "It's one of the key **elements** of an investigative program. The perfect soundtrack will really **enhance** the show!"

"Eh," Lucas said. "OK."

We had our jobs nailed down. Now we needed a concept for our first episode. And a title.

"Exposé titles are always **exaggerated**," I said. "That's how you get people to watch."

I gave the example of "Confessions of a Guilty Grandma," the Purse Lady show.

"The title made me want to know what the grandma was guilty of!" I said.

I had come up with a bunch of possible titles for our first episode. I wrote them down on my dry-erase **easel**.

"BLADDERS GONE BERSERK!"
"UNDER SUSPICION: KIDS WHO LEAK"
"CLOGGED: THE RECTUM REPORT"

Lucas rolled his eyes. Not the best **etiquette**, a.k.a. manners. Apparently, he was not **enamored** with my ideas.

I erased that last one. I didn't think anyone would want to watch a show with the word rectum in the title. Then I jotted down a few more:

"ENCOPRESIS: SOLVED!"
"UROLOGY UNIT: UNDERCOVER"
"EXHIBIT A: ABDOMINAL X-RAY"

I actually had one more idea, but I wasn't going to write it down—yet. I knew Charlotte would like it, but I thought the idea might send Lucas sliding down the fire pole.

Because it was about enemas.

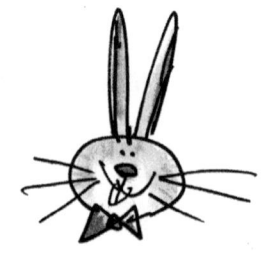

CHAPTER 15

At first, I gave myself an enema every **evening**, like Dr. Pooper had recommended. I did it between dinner and bath time. After a week, my poop accidents stopped. Entirely.

I almost couldn't believe it. I was **euphoric**—possibly the happiest I had ever been.

I mean, pee accidents were awful, but poop accidents were THE WORST. My life was already 100% better.

However, after a month, I was still having pee accidents. Not every day, like before. But still every single night.

Dr. Pooper had **encouraged** me to be patient, and I was trying my best. But honestly, after all that **enemizing**, I felt entitled to dry sheets! I felt I had **earned** it.

My frustration was **escalating**.

One night before bed, with my head resting on Ernest, I said, "Ernest, it's taking an **eternity**. Will I *ever* wake up dry?"

Discouraged, my mom and I went on another **excursion** to Dr. Pooper's office.

"Well, if it isn't Emma the **Emissary** to the Enema Empire!" Dr. Pooper said.

An emissary, FYI, is someone who's been sent somewhere important—like a royal messenger.

Then he said, "Say, what's new on your E list?"

"**Encumbered**," I replied. "I'm feeling weighed down. My enuresis is interfering with my life. I don't ever want to see a pull-up again."

Dr. Pooper **exuded** confidence.

"**Egads**! Emma. Considering where you started, your progress has **eclipsed** my **expectations**!"

Dr. Pooper said my rectum wasn't clogged anymore. Still, it needed more time to shrink back to normal size, regain its **elasticity**, and stop whacking out my bladder nerves.

"An enema is a marvelous tool, but it is not an **elixir**!" Dr. Pooper said.

Elixir was already on my E list. It means "magic potion."

Dr. Pooper told me it's normal for progress to

be **erratic**, a.k.a. inconsistent—to have a streak of dry days and then an accident. He also said it's hard to **estimate** how long it will take for enuresis to stop, since it's different for every kid.

"Just keep on pooping!" he said. "Keep launching those torpedoes!"

Dr. Pooper said my goal should be to poop twice a day: once after my enema and one extra time, too. On some days, I could do that. But other days, I couldn't.

To **expedite** my progress, a.k.a. speed things up, Dr. Pooper recommended I take **Ex-Lax**, chocolate squares with medicine inside.

I started Ex-Lax the next day.

The medicine gave me cramps, but escalated my pooping. In my estimation, 1.) cramping was better than constipation, and 2.) the chocolate squares didn't taste half bad.

Soon, I could feel when I needed to poop and pee. My signals were working again, at least during the day. I even started using the bathrooms at school and at Food 4 Even Less.

I was a pooping machine!

In fact, at my next appointment, Dr. Pooper called me Her **Eminence**, Emma the Excavator.

"I suggest you put *eminence* in your notebook," Dr. Pooper said. "It means a 'person of high rank.' You rank high, Emma!"

A few minutes later, he called me Emma of the **Empty** Eisenhower Expressway, which he told me is also known as the Ike.

"You're like the Ike at **eleven** p.m. on **Easter**," he said. "Entirely empty!"

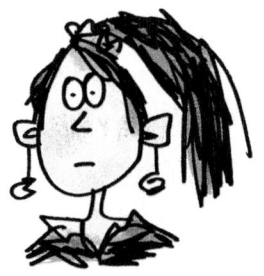

CHAPTER 16

The day after our E Club meeting, Lucas didn't talk to me at school. Actually, he didn't talk to me for three days straight. But he wasn't totally avoiding me, either—not like before.

One morning at recess, right before zombie tag, I whispered, "Tomorrow. Treehouse. Four o'clock."

I wasn't sure if Lucas would tell his mom about the meeting, so after school, I asked my mom to call his mom and tell Lucas I was going to make cinnamon-sugar popcorn. I thought that might be an **enticement.**

By 4:07 the next afternoon (according to my potty watch), Lucas still had not shown up at the treehouse. Charlotte and I were feeling dejected.

We were munching on the popcorn when, finally, we heard footsteps on the ladder.

Lucas had decided to come after all!

"I heard there's popcorn," Lucas said, as he poked his head through the beaded curtain.

"I roasted it with cinnamon and sugar!" I said, handing him a big bowl.

Now that Lucas was back, I was feeling bold and **energized.**

"Hey, guys," I said. "I invented a new word!"

Charlotte and Lucas weren't surprised. Everyone at school knows I'm a word enthusiast.

I've won the spelling bee three years in a row, and most kids know about my E notebook, since I wear it at school.

"Oh yeah?" Charlotte said. "What's the word?"

"*Enemizing.* It means giving yourself an enema."

"Cool!" Charlotte said. "I'm an expert at enemizing."

Lucas winced, the way I do when I get my flu shot.

"Well, *I'm* not enemizing," he said. "Not ever."

"That's fine, Lucas," Charlotte said.

"Dr. Pooper loves my word!" I continued. "He said he's going to use it with his patients. Maybe it will become a real word, like in the dictionary!"

That could totally happen. Did you know new words get added to the dictionary every year? Language **evolves** over time, and the dictionary is always **expanding**. Every year, dictionary **executives** vote to add new words—words that previously did not exist but now are used **extensively**.

For example, *selfie* was added about ten years before I was born. *Bestie* was added when I was a baby. Maybe *enemize* will be next!

I decided to tell Charlotte and Lucas my idea for the first episode of our exposé.

I wrote the title on my easel: "The Mysterious Case of the Bedwetting Boy."

"Intriguing!" Charlotte said.

Lucas was **expressionless**. And silent.

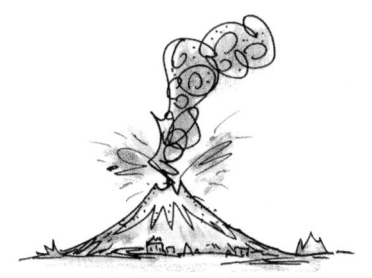

CHAPTER 17

I kept up my enemas and my Ex-Lax, and eventually my daytime accidents stopped. I started wearing underwear to school. That was huge. That was amazing.

Then one morning, for the first time in my entire **existence**, I woke up with a dry pull-up. I wasn't **expecting** that turn of **events**, so I checked three times to ensure it was actually true.

I was **ebullient**—all smiles.

Instead of bounding out of bed, I relaxed for a while, **ensconced** in my soft, fluffy comforter. I wanted to savor the **enormity** of what had happened. It was a big deal.

"Boy, Ernest," I said. "This is the life, eh?"

That morning will be **eternally etched** in my mind.

Eventually, I hopped out of bed and delivered the news to my parents. My dad **erupted** into applause. My mom burst into tears. We called Grandma, and later that day, we all celebrated at the pastry shop, with chocolate-iced éclairs.

Now I wake up dry every day. I even wear underwear to bed. I only enemize twice a week, and soon my enema treatment will end entirely.

That **era** will be over.

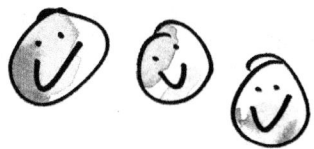

CHAPTER 18

I knew why Lucas wasn't enthused about the idea of "The Mysterious Case of the Bedwetting Boy": he thought the Bedwetting Boy was *him*.

But it wasn't. Of course not.

I explained to Charlotte and Lucas that the Bedwetting Boy in the title was actually a five-year-old kid Dr. Pooper once told me about.

The boy grew up in the 1980s. FYI, that was before texting, **emailing**, and **emojis**. Before cellphones, even. Back then, your phone had to be plugged into a wall! In my estimation, 1.) a phone you can't carry around seems useless, and 2.) the world must have been a difficult place in the 1980s.

Anyway, the Bedwetting Boy, who grew up in Canada, was the first kid in the world, at least the first we know of, whose enuresis was fixed with enemas.

"His dad was a doctor, named Dr. O'Regan," I explained, "Dr. O'Regan invented the idea of using enemas to stop accidents, and it worked!"

Lucas rolled his eyes.

Charlotte, on the other hand, was **entranced** by the story, a.k.a. super interested.

Charlotte has always been **enthralled** by inventions and **experiments**. She's already finished her **entry** for the next Invention

Convention. It's called the Bathtub Book Hook. A pulley hangs from a hook on your bathtub wall and clips onto your book, **enabling** you to read without worrying that your book might fall into the water. To turn the pages, you press a button that activates a claw.

Clever, eh? And well **executed**, too! I know because I tested it out with *Harry Potter and the Order of the Phoenix*, the heaviest Harry Potter book.

Anyway, I was telling you about the Bedwetting Boy. Back in the 1980s, his dad accomplished something **extraordinary**: He proved, in a series of scientific experiments, that constipation—not "bad behavior" or stress or deep sleep—causes enuresis and encopresis.

"Dr. O'Regan also proved enemas could stop accidents!" I said.

Lucas rolled his eyes again.

I handed Charlotte and Lucas the script I had written for "The Mysterious Case of the Bedwetting Boy."

Here's an **excerpt**, a.k.a. a short section.

FADE IN:

THE CAMERA ZOOMS IN ON A MAP OF CANADA

        CHARLOTTE [VOICE OVER]
The year was 1983.

The place: Montreal, Canada.

The home of Dr. Sean O'Regan, a hardworking doctor, husband, and father of three boys.

CAMERA ZOOMS IN ON A PHOTO OF THE O'REGAN FAMILY

The O'Regan household was a happy one.

But something was amiss: The middle son, age five, was wetting his bed. Every night. Sometimes twice.

CAMERA ZOOMS IN ON THE MIDDLE SON

Often, the boy would wake his parents. Mrs. O'Regan, sound asleep, would **elbow** her husband to help their son change his sheets and pajamas.

Because of his accidents, the O'Regan boy did not want to go on vacations. He didn't want to sleep anywhere but home.

His enuresis was causing tension in the family.

"You're a doctor, for heaven's sake," Mrs. O'Regan told her husband. "Can't you do something?"

But Dr. O'Regan was stumped.

Back then, most doctors believed

that children wet their beds on purpose—that children with enuresis were misbehaving.

Dr. O'Regan did not believe that. He felt that assumption was unfair.

Unproven.

Untrue.

But the mystery persisted. What was causing the boy's accidents? What was the culprit?

These questions troubled Dr. O'Regan. They gnawed at him.

Until one day, Dr. O'Regan discovered the truth.

CUE SUSPENSFUL MUSIC

The discovery not only changed his son's life but also changed medical history.

CAMERA CUTS TO CHARLOTTE, WEARING A TRENCH COAT AND STANDING OUTSIDE AT DUSK, IN THE SHADOWS

I'm Charlotte, your host, and a fourth grader at Eastside Elementary.

On tonight's episode of "Constipation Investigation: The Untold Story!" we will **explore** "The Mysterious Case of the Bedwetting Boy."

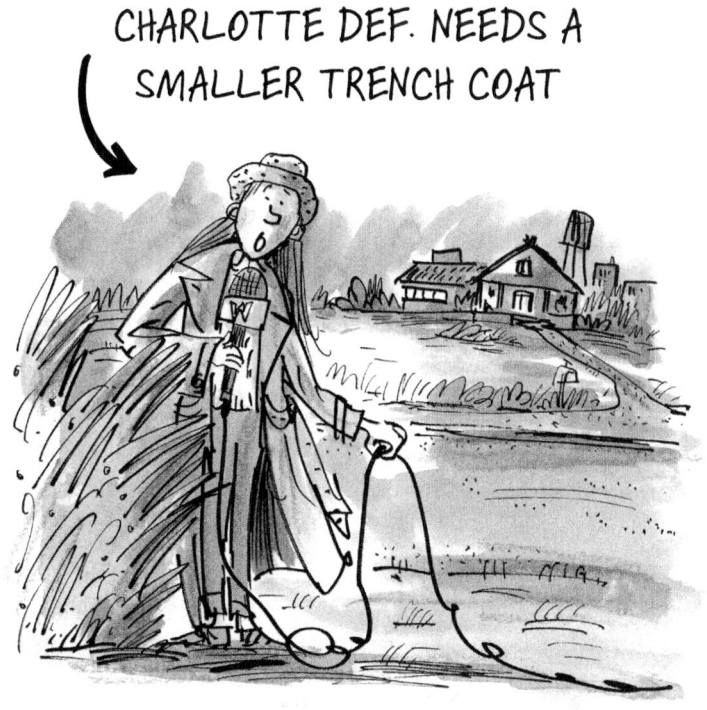

CHARLOTTE DEF. NEEDS A SMALLER TRENCH COAT

```
What you are about to watch is
one hundred percent true.

No names have been changed.

No facts have been altered.

Stay with us.
```

"Awesome!" Charlotte said.

"Can you pass the popcorn?" Lucas said.

———

A few days later, my mom drove Charlotte, Lucas, and me to Dr. Pooper's office to interview him for our episode.

Dr. Pooper told us that Dr. O'Regan was retired and not available for filming, but Dr. Pooper knew all about "The Mysterious Case of the Bedwetting Boy" and was excited to appear on camera. He promised us an "**exclusive**," not that anyone else wanted to interview him.

"Enchanted to assist you and your esteemed **entourage**, Emma!" Dr. Pooper said. "You and your **exemplary** associates are going to change the world! You have my **everlasting** gratitude!"

By now, you are aware of Dr. Pooper's **eccentricities**, a.k.a. his peculiarities. I mean, he took his shoe and sock off during my appointment. He thinks a purple goldfish tie matches a blue and white striped shirt!

I worried about what might happen if Dr. Pooper spoke **extemporaneously** on camera, a.k.a. without rehearsing. Who knew what silliness might **emanate** from his mouth?

Before his on-air interview, I sat Dr. Pooper down for a talk. I told him we planned to use his real name, not Dr. Pooper. And I **exhorted**, a.k.a. begged, him not to remove his socks or his shoes or even his **eyeglasses** and definitely not to say "chop a log" or "chocolate hot dog."

"'Constipation Investigation' is an exposé," I reminded him. "Not a fifth-grade Halloween party."

"Fear not, Emma!" Dr. Pooper replied. "I will be the **epitome** of **earnestness**. The picture of professionalism!"

And . . . he was. I was relieved.

Charlotte wore her mom's trench coat and looked like a real TV investigator. Well, the coat was too big, but we had to **economize**, a.k.a. save money.

———

A few days later, I showed the episode to my mom, right before our E Club meeting. She said the writing sounded professional. "Emma, you could get hired on *Forensic Files II!*" she said.

Charlotte 100% had a talent for hosting. She

spoke **emphatically**—in a convincing voice—while her **expressive** face **evinced emotion**. She showed that she truly cared about the story.

    Our meeting was about to start, so I headed over to the treehouse.

    "Have a great meeting!" my mom said. "Dad's in the kitchen. I'll be on the elliptical!"

    "Sure, Mom," I said.

    I wasn't exactly shocked when she added, "Or, I might run some **errands**!"

    At the meeting, all of us watched the episode I had **edited**.

    "Not bad," Lucas said.

    For Lucas, that was a big compliment. Lucas isn't one to **embellish**, a.k.a. say more than is necessary.

    Amazingly, Lucas didn't even roll his eyes.

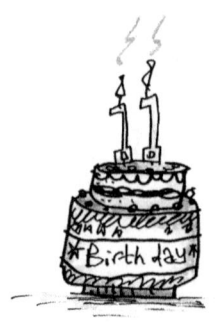

EPILOGUE

FYI an **epilogue** is an **ending** that catches you up on what's happened since the main story concluded.

I have a *lot* of news to report, so I'm going to **encapsulate**, a.k.a. summarize, it here.

For one thing, "Constipation Investigation: The Untold Story!" has become **enormously** popular.

I was right. A catchy title **entices** viewers! Dozens of parents have posted comments about the episode.

I'm going to share three comments that were especially **edifying**—comments that made me feel like the E Club is making a difference.

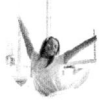 **grateful mom** Dear E Club. You kids changed our family's life! It wasn't until I watched your show that I realized our daughter was not purposefully ignoring the urge to poop. She wasn't even feeling it! I wish I'd known that earlier. I used to scold her, even though I tried not to. I apologized, and she accepted my apology. She is doing enemas now, and her accidents have stopped! She is a different kid than she was a year ago. Before, she was anxious and sad. Now she smiles all the time!

One mom posted a video of a marble run that her son had **engineered** for a third-grade project. It was called TOBY'S DIGESTIVE SYSTEM and was made from cereal boxes, paper plates, and toilet paper rolls.

Toby's mom wrote: "Because of the E Club, my son made this amazing marble run!"

On the video, Toby drops a marble into

the "mouth." As the marble rolls down the **esophagus**, into the stomach, and then into the colon and rectum, Toby offers his commentary:

"Look at all this hard poop! This rectum is clogged. It's constipated! But that's okay, I'll just give it an enema!"

Another mom posted:

J.L.B.'s mom To the E Club kids:
My son J.L.B. had three poop accidents at his sixth birthday party at a park. Poor guy! Even after that, we kept giving him poop powder. But when I showed my son your video, he said, "Enema! Enema! Enema!" The next day, he tried his first enema and felt so much better. Now he sings, "I just can't wait for my enema" to the Lion King song! His accidents have stopped, and soon he'll be done with enemas. Keep up your investigations!
P.S. Charlotte needs a trench coat that fits.

Oh, I need to update you about that, too. Charlotte's mom was so excited about our show that she bought Charlotte a coat that fits perfectly.

Dr. Pooper was super **encouraging**, too. Last time I visited his office, he said, "Well, if it isn't Emma the **Envoy** to the Enema **Embassy**!"

I added *embassy* to my E list (along with lots of other new words!). An embassy is, basically, an important office. I think Dr. Pooper's office is important because that's where lots of kids learn about enemas.

I also added *envoy* to my list. Dr. Pooper said it means "a messenger on a mission."

I definitely feel like I'm on a mission: to help other kids with enuresis or encopresis feel brave enough to try enemas.

It's not an easy mission. I know enemas **evoke** strong **emotions**. In my estimation, adults assume that enemas are 1.) **"excessive,"** a.k.a. unnecessary, and 2.) more than kids can handle.

I disagree! Some kids really do need them.

And if I can enemize, anyone can.

I have a lot more to update you on. I bet you're wondering if Lucas ever tried an enema. Well, he did.

Eventually, his opposition **eroded**, a.k.a. wore down. I think he got tired of having accidents and realized that poop powder wasn't working for him.

Lucas doesn't like to talk about his enuresis, but he's going to basketball sleepaway camp this summer, so I know his treatment is going well.

Charlotte, Lucas, and I have **embarked** on the second episode of "Constipation Investigation: The Untold Story!" I'm not going to reveal the title just yet.

If you have ideas for future episodes, we'd love to hear them.

Probably the biggest news is that I'm eleven now, and my birthday party was a sleepover!

Jasmine came, and so did three other girls from our class. We lined up our sleeping bags in the basement, really close together, right next to the elliptical.

"I guess I won't be exercising tonight!" my mom said.

"I guess not," I replied.

In the morning, from inside my sleeping bag, I checked to ensure my underwear was dry. I still do that sometimes, even though I haven't had an accident in forever.

My underwear *was* dry, as dry as my T-shirt. But my eyes weren't. I could feel a few tears welling up—tears of **elation**, a.k.a. 100% pure happiness. I couldn't believe I was hosting a slumber party. I had dreamed about it for so long.

My friends were still sleeping, so they didn't see me cry.

Ernest was my only **eyewitness**.

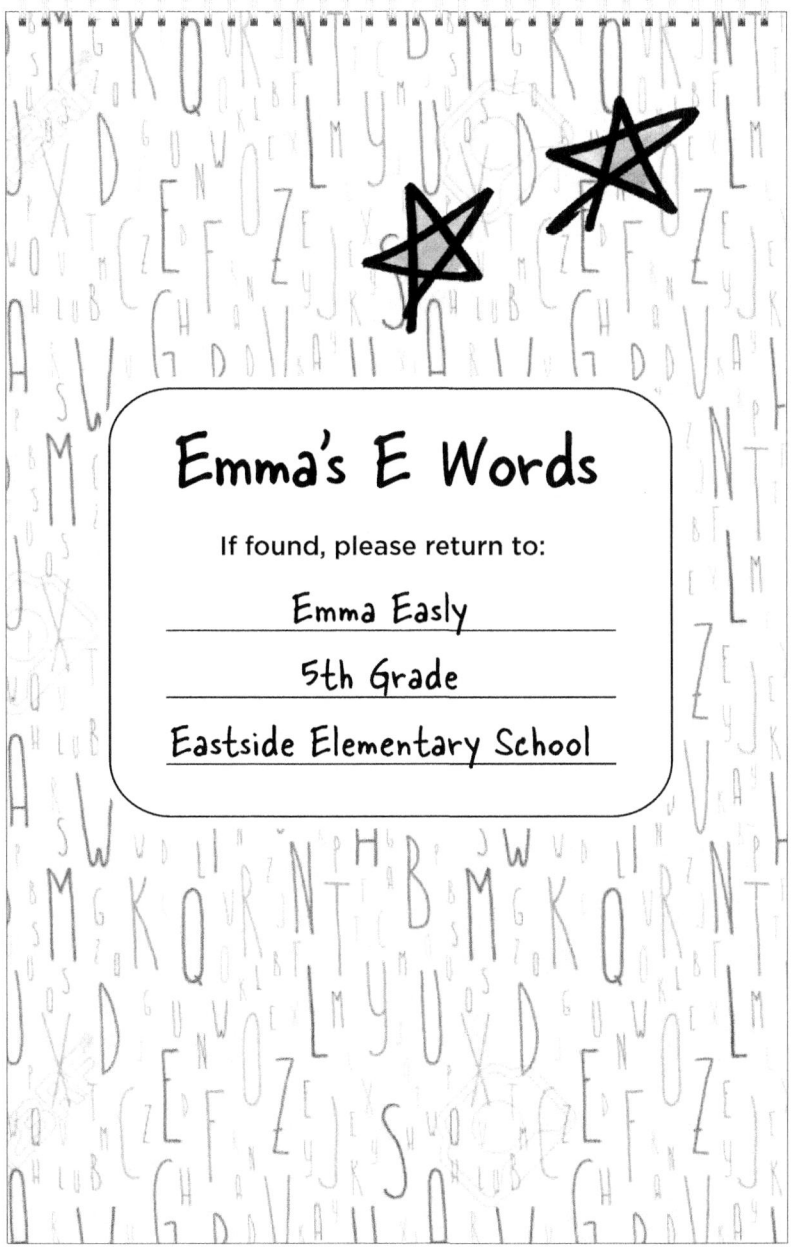

	623.	executive
	624.	entirely
	625.	expect
★	626.	enuresis — pee accidents
	627.	either
★	628.	encopresis — poop accidents
	629.	even
	630.	embarrassing
	631.	episodes
	632.	error
	633.	everywhere
	634.	except
	635.	evidently
	636.	extrovert
	637.	elect
	638.	enjoy
★	639.	excel — to be really good at something
	640.	exaggeration
	641.	endlessly
	642.	entertained
	643.	example
	644.	easily
	645.	effort
	646.	eight-letter
	647.	excellent
★	648.	employed — hired for a job
	649.	essayist
	650.	expresses
★	651.	estimation — opinion
	652.	edible
	653.	exaggerates
	654.	exercises
★	655.	emulating — copying
	656.	English
★	657.	extended — lengthened
	658.	eyes
	659.	enormous
	660.	encounter
	661.	enter
★	662.	essentially — basically
★	663.	enema — squeezy tube w/ medicine to help you poop
	664.	exactly

112

	665.	enemas
☆	666.	emphatic — definite, forceful in your opinion
	667.	established
☆	668.	extensive — big/long
☆	669.	etc. — and so on (short for etcetera)
☆	670.	en route — on the way
	671.	encountered
☆	672.	eminent — famous, well known
	673.	edge
☆	674.	enables — allows
	675.	entire
☆	676.	egotistical — braggy
	677.	eyed
	678.	exact
	679.	exercising
	680.	exchanged
	681.	expressions
☆	682.	emboldened — confident
☆	683.	epiphany — sudden inspiration
☆	684.	endorsed — approved
	685.	entered
☆	686.	erect — to build
	687.	epic
☆	688.	edifice — building
☆	689.	equivalent — about equal
	690.	equal
☆	691.	Eiffel Tower
	692.	Empire State Building
	693.	elaborate
	694.	elegant
	695.	expensive
	696.	Etsy
	697.	equipped
☆	698.	expeditiously — super fast
	699.	every
☆	700.	eligible — allowed to join
	701.	eager
	702.	expand
☆	703.	eradicate — get rid of
☆	704.	envision — imagine, predict
☆	705.	else
☆	706.	exposé — shocking report that uncovers the truth

113

☆ 707. earnings
708. extravagant — over-the-top fancy or expensive
☆ 709. exotic — unusual, far far away
710. existed
711. everyone
☆ 712. establishments — businesses
713. exciting
☆ 714. endeavor — pursuit, job
715. experience
☆ 716. excruciating — worse than painful
717. escape
718. Earth
719. exile
☆ 720. Europa — one of Jupiter's icy moons
721. exist
722. event
723. ever
724. enough
☆ 725. echoed
726. enlistee — person who joins a group
727. exceptionally
728. eureka — OMG!
729. embarrass
730. extra
731. eavesdrop
☆ 732. emanated — came from
☆ 733. enlist — to join
☆ 734. equitably — fairly
735. expected
736. exert
737. entrust
☆ 738. evasive — won't give you a straight answer
739. extraterrestrial
☆ 740. enigma — a mystery, problem you can't figure out
741. earthly
742. eggplant
743. eight

114

	744.	earning		761.	exams
☆	745.	explicitly — obviously, specifically	☆	762.	exerted — used (exerted myself = made an effort)
☆	746.	empathize — relate to			
☆	747.	extent — level, "to some extent" = partly	☆	763.	eluded — avoided, escaped
	748.	eye-rolling		764.	erupt
	749.	exclaimed		765.	eavesdropped
☆	750.	exasperated — super annoyed		766.	emerged
	751.	exception	☆	767.	engagement — commitment, appointment
☆	752.	egregiously — outrageously		768.	excuse
	753.	everything		769.	exposed
	754.	exhausted		770.	excluded
	755.	evenings		771.	excluding
☆	756.	éclairs — French pastries w/ cream inside and icing outside	☆	772.	eroding — wearing down
				773.	extra-large
				774.	elevated
	757.	erase		775.	escapes
	758.	episode	☆	776.	embezzled — stole
	759.	elephant		777.	empties
☆	760.	earnestly — seriously, with good intentions		778.	earbuds
				779.	encourages

	780.	Encyclopedia Brown — SILLY BOOKS!		803.	examination
				804.	elementary
☆	781.	expenses — costs	☆	805.	empathized — related to
	782.	especially	☆	806.	exacerbated — made worse
	783.	exposés		807.	environment
	784.	evidence		808.	emphasis
	785.	evaluate	☆	809.	ensure — make sure
☆	786.	erroneously — wrongly	☆	810.	exonerated — proven innocent
☆	787.	entrenched — stuck			
	788.	elliptical	☆	811.	enlightening — educational, interesting
	789.	exercise			
	790.	electric		812.	expression
	791.	easy	☆	813.	evolving — changing
	792.	eliminate		814.	eats
	793.	eagerly	☆	815.	eons — ages, forever
	794.	evaporate	☆	816.	emblazoned — decorated, illustrated
	795.	embarrassment			
☆	796.	expertise — skill	☆	817.	exterior — the outside of something
☆	797.	escalated — increased			
☆	798.	excrement — poop!		818.	emergency
☆	799.	excreta — poop!		819.	embroidered
	800.	ended	☆	820.	eccentric — weird, odd (like Dr. Pooper!)
☆	801.	enthusiast — fanatic			
☆	802.	erudite — knowledgeable	☆	821.	ensemble — outfit

	822.	examine
☆	823.	escorted — guided
	824.	equipment
☆	825.	elicited — produced, caused
☆	826.	earsplitting — insanely loud
☆	827.	expertly — with lots of skill
☆	828.	extracted — pulled out
	829.	entangled
☆	830.	extricated — removed
☆	831.	exhibited — showed
☆	832.	externally — on the outside
	833.	energy
☆	834.	electromagnetic — electric forces
	835.	end
☆	836.	Eisenhower Expressway — super crowded highway in Chicago (*never go there!)
☆	837.	ensnarled — totally stuck
	838.	explained
☆	839.	evacuate — to empty completely
☆	840.	essential — necessary, totally important
☆	841.	expel — push out, banish
	842.	excavator
	843.	embarrassed
☆	844.	eke (out) — to barely do something
☆	845.	excess — extra
	846.	expands
☆	847.	enchilada — YUM!
☆	848.	entitled — titled (like a chapter title) OR deserving
	849.	each
	850.	enlarged
☆	851.	encroaches (upon) — invades, intrudes
	852.	enthusiasm
☆	853.	eyeballs
☆	854.	ergo — therefore
	855.	experienced

117

☆ 856. expunged — removed,
   857. erased
   858. evil
   859. earthquake
☆ 860. edification — education
   861. education
   862. exhibition
   863. elastic
   864. endless
☆ 865. engrossed — super interested
   866. eye-popping
   867. earth-shaking
☆ 868. evaded — avoided
   869. elsewhere
☆ 870. evident — obvious
   871. excusable
   872. ecstatic
☆ 873. enunciating — pronouncing
   874. enemy
   875. entertain
   876. Etch A Sketch
   877. extreme
☆ 878. expelled — pushed out

☆ 879. extravaganza — big deal, awesome happening
☆ 880. Egyptians
   881. Egypt
☆ 882. esoteric — obscure, weird (stuff nobody else knows)
   883. Egyptian
   884. enjoyable
   885. employment
☆ 886. effective — useful, valuable
☆ 887. exempt — spared, released (like, you don't have to do it)
☆ 888. eclectic — diverse (you have a bunch of different things)
   889. eventually
☆ 890. enterprising — imaginative, creative and hardworking
   891. easier
☆ 892. estimable — decent, OK
☆ 893. efficacious — very useful

☆ 894. enumerated — numbered, counted
☆ 895. elated — super happy
896. ear ⟶ 🦻
☆ 897. exultant — thrilled, same as "elated"
☆ 898. endure — tolerate, deal with (something bad)
899. excited
900. easygoing
☆ 901. exhortation — advice
☆ 902. escapade — incident, happening
☆ 903. entreated — begged
☆ 904. enterprise — big project
☆ 905. equivocated — hesitated or refused to answer
906. enthusiastic
☆ 907. embarking — starting
908. eased
909. emphasized
☆ 910. embraced — accepted
☆ 911. empowered — encouraged and confident
☆ 912. envied — felt jealous
☆ 913. elected — chose
914. exited
915. exhale
☆ 916. endurable — bearable, like not as bad as you expected
☆ 917. ejected — burst out
918. explosive
919. eruption
920. expert
☆ 921. enemize — to give yourself an enema
922. effortlessly
☆ 923. enemizer — a person who gives themselves an enema
☆ 924. extraordinaire — excellent, awesome
☆ 925. excellency — a fancy title, like "Your Awesomeness"
☆ 926. esteemed — honored, appreciated

☆ 927. exalted — high-ranking, at the top
☆ 928. empress — title for a female ruler, like a queen
☆ 929. enchanted — delighted, happy
☆ 930. echelon — level
931. earlier
932. explain
☆ 933. eschewed — rejected, gave up
934. encourage
935. experiences
☆ 936. enthused — excited about
☆ 937. effusive — full of compliments
938. eventful
☆ 939. expounded — talked more about, gave more details about
940. exclamation
941. expose
942. explanations
943. extinct
☆ 944. enact — put into action (like, pass a law)
☆ 945. erroneous — mistaken
946. engine
☆ 947. enraged — super mad
948. educate
☆ 949. exposure — publicity
☆ 950. endorsement — approval, support
☆ 951. exuberant — super cheerful
952. energetic
☆ 953. eloquently — persuasively (used with speaking)
954. entertaining
☆ 955. editor — person who decides what information is important and what's not
956. expendable
957. Elvis
958. Eminem

120

	959.	effect	☆	978.	egads! — an old-person expression for surprise, like "Oh wow!"
☆	960.	elements — parts			
☆	961.	enhance — improve			
	962.	exaggerated			
	963.	easel	☆	979.	eclipsed — surpassed, exceeded
☆	964.	etiquette — manners			
☆	965.	enamored — approving, fond of		980.	expectations
			☆	981.	elasticity — bounciness, springiness
	966.	exhibit			
	967.	evening	☆	982.	elixir — magic potion
☆	968.	euphoric — super excited	☆	983.	erratic — inconsistent, unreliable
	969.	encouraged			
☆	970.	enemizing — giving yourself an enema		984.	estimate
			☆	985.	expedite — speed up
☆	971.	earned	☆	986.	Ex-Lax — chocolate squares of medicine that make you poop
☆	972.	escalating — increasing			
☆	973.	eternity — forever	☆	987.	eminence — greatness, importance (Your Eminence = Your Greatness)
☆	974.	excursion — a trip			
☆	975.	emissary — a messenger			
☆	976.	encumbered — burdened, weighed down		988.	empty
				989.	eleven
☆	977.	exuded — showed, displayed		990.	Easter

☆ 991. enticement — an incentive, like a bribe that motivates you to do something
992. energized
☆ 993. evolves — changes
994. expanding
☆ 995. executives — bosses
☆ 996. extensively — almost everywhere
997. expressionless
998. existence
999. expecting
1000 events
☆ 1001. ebullient — extra joyful
☆ 1002. ensconced — deeply settled, lodged, hidden
☆ 1003. enormity — hugeness
☆ 1004. eternally — forever
☆ 1005. etched — imprinted, stamped
☆ 1006. erupted — burst
1007. era
1008. emailing
1009. emojis
☆ 1010. entranced — so fascinated that you can't pay attention to anything else
☆ 1011. enthralled — extremely interested (like entranced, but happier)
1012. experiments
1013. entry
☆ 1014. enabling — allowing
1015. executed
1016. extraordinary
☆ 1017. excerpt — short part of a book, movie, video, TV show
1018. elbow
1019. explore
☆ 1020. exclusive — special, like only certain people are allowed

122

- ☆ 1021. entourage — posse, group that follows you around
- ☆ 1022. exemplary — so excellent that it's an example for others
- 1023. everlasting
- ☆ 1024. eccentricities — oddities, weirdness
- ☆ 1025. extemporaneously — without practicing
- ☆ 1026. emanate — come out of
- ☆ 1027. exhorted — encouraged, begged
- 1028. eyeglasses
- ☆ 1029. epitome — perfect example of
- ☆ 1030. earnestness — seriousness
- ☆ 1031. economize — save money
- ☆ 1032. emphatically — with strong feeling
- 1033. expressive
- ☆ 1034. evinced — showed
- 1035. emotion
- 1036. errands
- 1037. edited
- 1038. embellish
- 1039. epilogue
- 1040. ending
- ☆ 1041. encapsulate — summarize
- 1042. enormously
- ☆ 1043. entices — convinces
- ☆ 1044. edifying — satisfying
- ☆ 1045. engineered — designed
- 1046. esophagus
- 1047. encouraging
- ☆ 1048. envoy — messenger
- ☆ 1049. embassy — important office
- ☆ 1050. evoke — bring out, stir up
- 1051. emotions
- ☆ 1052. excessive — unnecessary
- ☆ 1053. eroded — wore down
- ☆ 1054. embarked — started
- ☆ 1055. elation — extreme happiness
- 1056. eyewitness

EMMA'S WORD GAMES

Here are some word games Dr. Pooper and I thought up.

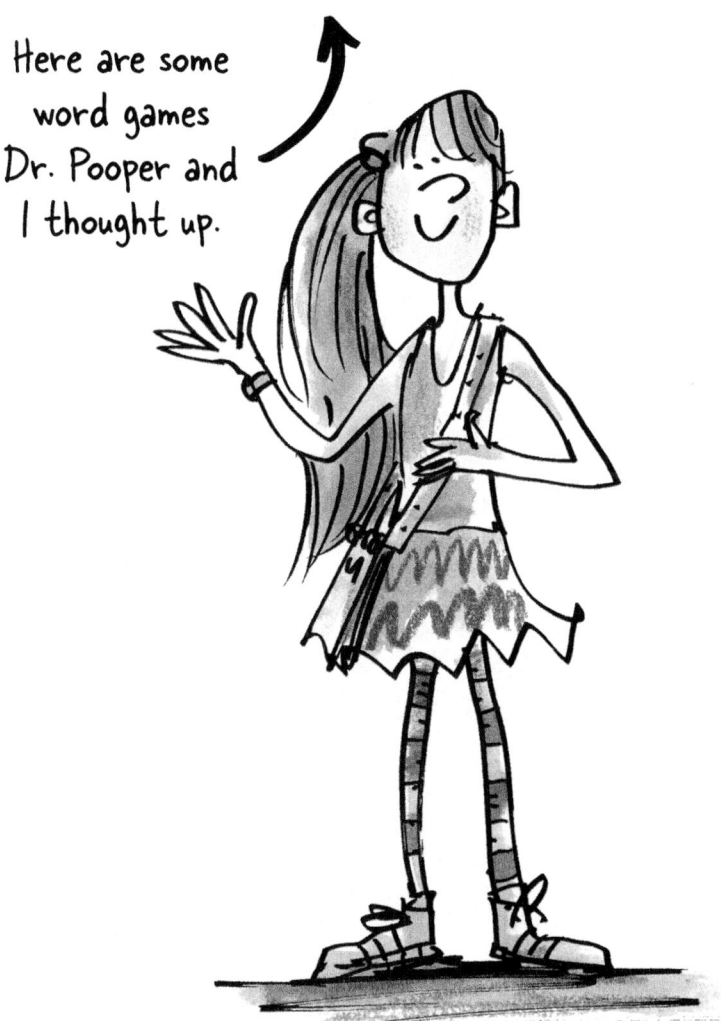

You can find lots more games and puzzles in
Dr. Pooper's Activity Book and Poop Calendar for Kids.

Find the Mystery Words

Each scrambled word below is a different shape of poop. First, unscramble the words. Then copy the shaded letters into the blanks to find the mystery words.

mshuum ___ ___ ___ ___ ___ ___

zefrno uyrogt ___ ___ ___ ___ ___ ___ ___ ___ ___ ___ ___

knase ___ ___ ___ ___ ___

ikmhklase ___ ___ ___ ___ ___ ___ ___ ___

wcotpyat ___ ___ ___ ___ ___ ___ ___ ___

pgdudin ___ ___ ___ ___ ___ ___ ___

glo ___ ___ ___

sbblo ___ ___ ___ ___ ___

sellpet ___ ___ ___ ___ ___ ___ ___

Mystery words: ___ ___ ___ ___ ___   ___ ___ ___ ___

(Hint: This is the best kind of poop!)

WORDFINDER

How many words can you make out of **ENEMA**?

2-letter words: _____ _____

_____ _____

3-letter words: _____ _____

4-letter words: _____ _____

_____ _____

Word Search: *Shapes of Poop*

Find all these different shapes of poop!
The words go across, down, and diagonally.

Milkshake	Pudding	Pebbles	Swirl
Frozen Yogurt	Log	Marbles	Hot Dog
Thin Snake	Mushy Blobs	Gravy	Walnuts
Hummus	Pellets	Diarrhea	Fluffy Cloud
Cow Patty	Lumpy Sausage	Rocks	Soft Mound

```
K X D N U O M T F O S H B D M U U W Q Y
V W M Z N Z H N P X O E F I P A O D K H
C P C H U M M U S T W R Y A V N D E Z M
C O G X O D D Z D E O D H R B Z A K H A
N D W L M C F O D Z A N L R N M B A L D
Q E V P T W G N E S S O W H R L Z H Y Q
J R S V A C S N M I I S X E R L K S E G
B W B J N T Y F F D F F J A U L J K N L
X A M Y A O T N L L Q D O M D H A L P L
I L Q P G D C Y U F L G P E G N K I R A
X N Z U G Y G F J R L Y P A S R N M U G
M U R G H T F B I G S F P N T E A B D I
V T P C M Y W W D A G A I C T V I V J T
H S T U C A S G U D W H X N X L S J Y H
Y V P L D A R S Y N T K R G O L M E M D
U H O S D D A B M U S H Y B L O B S G H
S U Z C T G I H L Q S T E L L E P X D F
D C G H E G R N C E T A P E B B L E S E
V O Z R L I G F G S S V W J M M O H Q K
S K Q I K F I V R O C K S L Y U R L W Q
```

127

DECODE THE MESSAGE

High five! You decoded the message!

Use the decoder to read this important message from Dr. Pooper.

D A O E P R Y V

WORDFINDER

How many words can you make out of **RECTUM**?

3-letter words: _____ _____ _____ _____

_____ _____ _____

4-letter words: _____ _____ _____

_____ _____ _____

128

CHANGE ONE LETTER!

Change one letter in each word to create a word related to your digestive system.

For example:
PROP —> change the "r" to "o" —> POOP

month
phew
tenth
jelly
color
rectus
ants
toiler

WHAT DID DR. POOPER SAY?

Cross out all the lower-case letters, g's and j's to find out what Dr. Pooper says about accidents. Then copy the letters into the message below.

A g C j g C I r D E m J N G T o S
j x w J m A g g o R J j p G E n l
G J N o p m O n j g J x q z e J T
i p G J y Y s a J O t m U G j x R
t o a J g F l m G A e U w L o T j

___ ___ ___ ___ ___ ___ ___ ___

___ ___ ___ ___   ___ ___ ___ ___

___ ___ ___ ___ ___   ___ ___ ___ ___ ___

WORDFINDER

How many words can you make out of **ENURESIS** (not including plurals)?

2-letter words: _____ _____ _____

3-letter words: _____ _____ _____ _____
_____ _____ _____ _____
_____ _____

4-letter words: _____ _____ _____
_____ _____ _____
_____ _____ _____
_____ _____

5-letter words: _____ _____ _____
_____ _____ _____
_____ _____ _____
_____ _____ _____

6-letter words: _____ _____

7-letter words: _____ _____

Rhyme It!

How many words can you rhyme with **BLADDER**?

_____ _____ _____

130

WORDFINDER

How many words can you make out of **ENCOPRESIS** (not including plurals)?

2-letter words:

3-letter words:

4-letter words:

5-letter words:

6-letter words:

7-letter words:

8-letter words:

Find the Mystery Words

Unscramble these bathroom words. Then, transfer the shaded letters to spell an important message about using the bathroom!

ulfhs ___ ___ [ ] ___

aosp [ ] ___ ___ ___

epe ___ ___ [ ]

kins [ ] ___ ___ ___

oppo ___ ___ [ ] ___

litteo rappe ___ ___ [ ] ___ ___ ___ ___ ___ ___ ___

eppar wleot ___ ___ ___ ___ ___ ___ [ ] ___ ___ ___

Mystery words: ___ ___   ___ ___ ___ ___

Rhyme It!

How many words can you rhyme with **POOP**?

_____ _____ _____ _____

_____ _____ _____ _____

Rhyme It!

How many words can you rhyme with **FLOPPY**?

_____ _____ _____ _____

UNCOVER A MESSAGE

Cross out all the lower-case letters, s's and p's to reveal where in your body your poop is most likely to get stuck. Then copy the letters into the message below.

**x e r I v q n N o w S P z b
n I r Y S O c b U z P c R S
q i R p E d P S C T u U z M**

___ ___ ___ ___ ___ ___ ___ ___ ___ ___ ___

WORDFINDER

How many words can you make out of **STRETCHED**?

5-letter words: _____ _____ _____

_____ _____ _____

_____ _____ _____

_____ _____ _____

_____ _____ _____

_____ _____ _____

_____ _____ _____

6-letter words: _____ _____

_____ _____

_____ _____

_____ _____

_____ _____

_____ _____

133

CROSSWORD:
FOLLOW YOUR FOOD!

Use the clues to fill in the puzzle.
The words relate to how your body makes poop and pee.

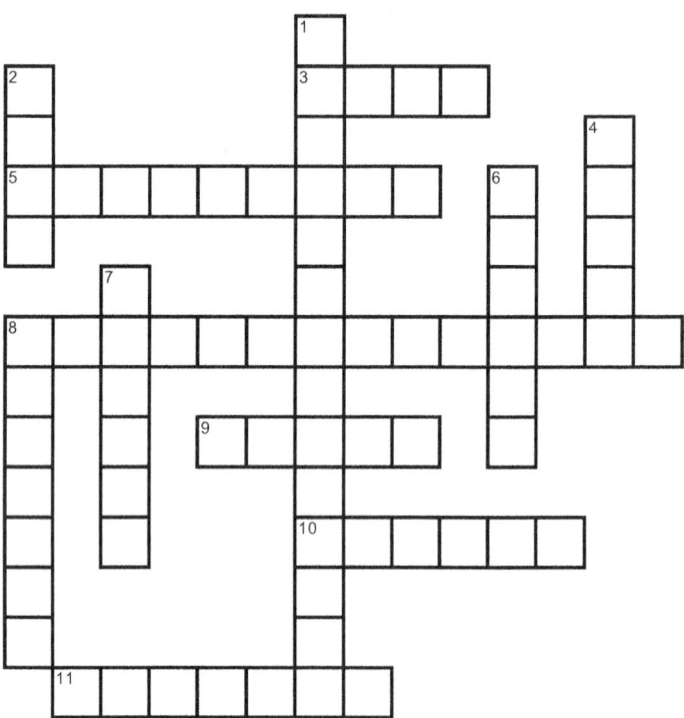

Across:
3. Your body's "exit door" for poop
5. Food slides down this tube to get to your stomach
8. The longest organ in your body
9. Needed for chomping!
10. It moves food around your mouth
11. It gets squished when your rectum is stuffed with poop

Down:
1. Where poop forms
2. You need teeth to do this
4. Another name for large intestine
6. Where poop piles up if you don't let it out
7. Liquid in your mouth that breaks down food
8. Where your food lands after you swallow it

WORDFINDER

How many words can you make out of **BLADDER**?

2-letter words: _____ _____

3-letter words: _____ _____ _____ _____
_____ _____ _____ _____
_____ _____ _____ _____
_____ _____ _____ _____

4-letter words: _____ _____ _____
_____ _____ _____
_____ _____ _____
_____ _____ _____
_____ _____ _____
_____ _____ _____

5-letter words: _____ _____ _____
_____ _____ _____
_____ _____ _____

Rhyme It!

How many words can you rhyme with **STOOL**?

_____ _____ _____ _____
_____ _____ _____ _____
_____ _____ _____ _____

All Over the World

Children all over the world — including the countries in this word search — have enuresis and encopresis
The words go across, downward, and diagonally.

Australia	Egypt	India	Japan	Russia
Brazil	France	Ireland	Kenya	Spain
Canada	Germany	Israel	Mexico	Sweden
China	Greece	Italy	Norway	Switzerland

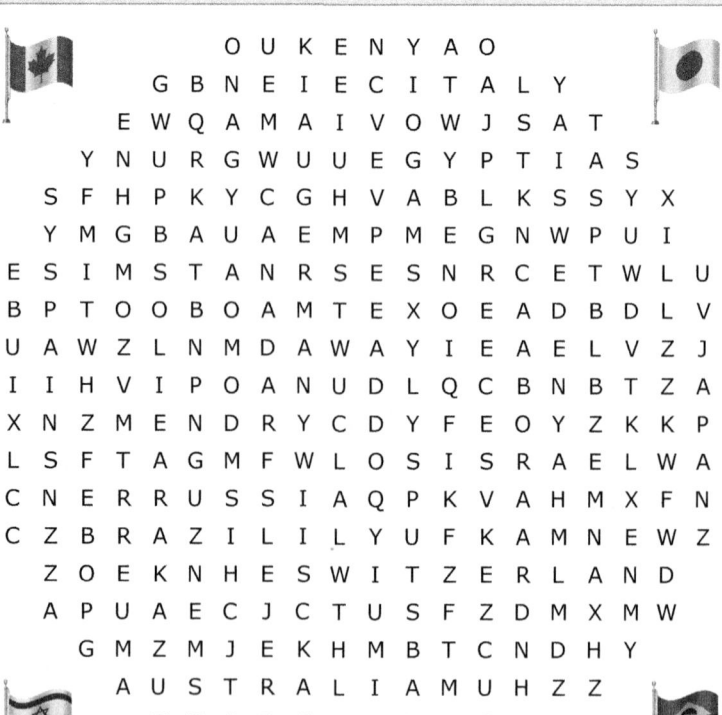

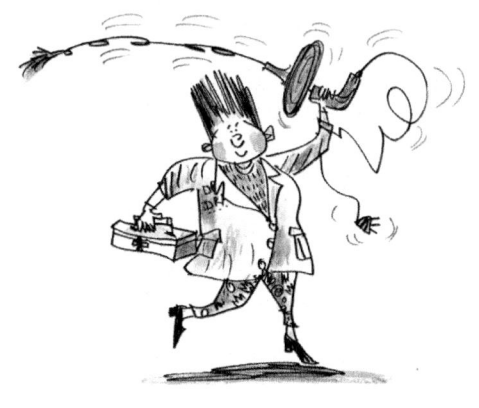

WORD GAME ANSWERS

page 126

MYSTERY WORDS: Mushy poop

UNSCRAMBLED WORDS:
hummus, frozen yogurt, snake, milkshake, cow patty, pudding, log, blobs, pellets

WORDFINDER: Possible words in ENEMA:
2-letter words: me, an, ma, am
3-letter words: men, man
4-letter words: name, mean, mane, amen

page 127

WORD SEARCH: SHAPES OF POOP

```
K X D N U O M T F O S H B D M U U W Q Y
V W M Z N Z H N P X O E F I P A O D K H
C P C H U M M U S T W R Y A V N D E Z M
C O G X O D D Z D E O D H R B Z A K H A
N D W L M C F O D Z A N L R N M B A L D
Q E V P T W G N E S S O W H R L Z H Y Q
J R S V A C S N M I I S X E R L K S E G
B W B J N T Y F F D F F J A U L J K N L
X A M Y A O T N L L Q D O M D H A L P L
I L Q P G D C Y U F L G P E G N K I R A
X N Z U G Y G F J R L Y P A S R N M U G
M U R G H T F B I G S F P N T E A B D I
V T P C M Y W W D A G A I C T V I V J T
H S T U C A S G U D W H X N X L S J Y H
Y V P L D A R S Y N T K R G O L M E M D
U H O S D D A B M U S H Y B L O B S G H
S U Z C T G I H L Q S T E L L E P X D F
D C G H E G R N C E T A P E B B L E S E
V O Z R L I G F G S S V W J M M O H Q K
S K Q I K F I V R O C K S L Y U R L W Q
```

page 128

DECODE THE MESSAGE:
Poop every day

WORDFINDER:
Possible words in RECTUM:
3-letter words: cue, rum, rut, met, emu, rue, cut
4-letter words: cute, cure, term, curt, true, ecru, mute

page 129

CHANGE ONE LETTER:
month > mouth
phew > chew
tenth > teeth
jelly > belly
color > colon
rectus > rectum
ants > anus
toiler > toilet

WHAT DID DR. POOPER SAY?
Right after you eat

page 130

WORDFINDER:
Possible words in ENURESIS:
2-letter words: us, in, is
3-letter words: sue, sun, urn, use, sin, rue, run, see, sir, ire
4-letter words: sine, user, urns, sure, sire, sere, rise, ruin, seen, seer, ruse
5-letter words: reuse, rinse, sense, risen, resin, issue, sneer, inure, urine, ensue, siren, reins, sinus, nurse
6-letter words: series, ensure
7-letter words: reissue, sunrise

RHYME IT!: BLADDER
Possible rhymes: ladder, madder, sadder

139

page 131

WORDFINDER: Possible words in ENCOPRESIS:
2-letter words: or, no, so, in, on, is
3-letter words: pee, son, pin, con, pie, per, cop, pen, pro, ice, one, rip, nip, see, nor, ire, ion, sip, sir, eon, sin, ore
4-letter words: seep, seen, epic, icon, see, iron, cope, cons, cone, coin, spin, crop, snip, corn, core, sore, ones, peon, rise, once, ripe, open, rice, peer, pier, nope, nice, pore, rose, ripe, rope, nose, pose
5-letter words: spice, price, scorn, press, poser, spine, score, spire, sneer, snipe, since, rinse, ripen, scene, scope, prose, sense, snore, scone, prone, poise, cross, opine, creep, crepe, crisp, piece, niece, noise
6-letter words: screen, nosier, person, prince, recipe, reopen, pierce, opener, prison, recess, corpse, censor, copier, sensor, senior, encore
7-letter words: process, sincere, pioneer, precise, species
8-letter words: princess, response

page 132

MYSTERY WORDS:
Use Soap

RHYME IT!: FLOPPY
Possible rhymes: copy, poppy, choppy, sloppy

RHYME IT! POOP
Possible rhymes: coop, coupe, croup, droop, dupe, goop, group, hoop, loop, scoop, snoop, soup, stoop, swoop, troop, troupe, whoop

page 133

UNCOVER A MESSAGE: In your rectum
WORDFINDER:
Possible words in STRETCHED:
5-letter words: teeth, retch, heeds, shred, sheet, sheer, steed, reeds, steer, reset, herds, these, three, crest, creed, chest, cheer, there, deter, erect, terse
6-letter words: street, detest, detect, desert, tether, etched, tested, secret, cheers, rested, screed, setter

page 134

CROSSWORD:
FOLLOW YOUR FOOD

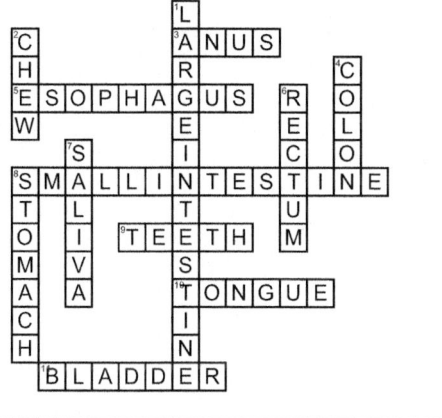

page 135

WORDFINDER:
Possible words in BLADDER:
2-letter words: ad, be
3-letter words: lad, lab, are, red, ale, led, rad, add, era, bad, bar, bed, ear, dad, dab, bra
4-letter words: bred, read, real, drab, earl, dear, dead, lard, dare, lead, bale, bald, bard, bare, bead, bear, able, bled, deal
5-letter words: blare, dared, bared, blade, bread, beard, dread, addle, alder

RHYME IT! STOOL
Possible rhymes:
cool, cruel, drool, dual, fool, fuel, ghoul, jewel, mule, pool, rule, school, spool, tool, yule

page 136

WORD SEARCH:
ALL OVER THE WORLD

```
            O U K E N Y A O
          G B N E I E C I T A L Y
          E W Q A M A I V O W J S A T
          Y N U R G W U U E G Y P T I A S
        S F H P K Y C G H V A B L K S S Y X
        Y M G B A U A E M P M E G N W P U I
      E S I M S T A N R S E S N R C E T W L U
      B P T O O B O A M T E X O E A D B D L V
      U A W Z L N M D A W A Y I E A E L V Z J
      I I H V I P O A N U D L Q C B N B T Z A
      X N Z M E N D R Y C D Y F E O Y Z K K P
      L S F T A G M F W L O S I S R A E L W A
      C N E R R U S S I A Q P K V A H M X F N
      C Z B R A Z I L I L Y U F K A M N E W Z
      Z O E K N H E S W I T Z E R L A N D
      A P U A E C J C T U S F Z D M X M W
        G M Z M J E K H M B T C N D H Y
          A U S T R A L I A M U H Z Z
          T W I R E L A N D S H Z
              N I I N D I A H
```

141

OTHER BOOKS FOR CHILDREN
by Suzanne Schlosberg and Steve Hodges, M.D.

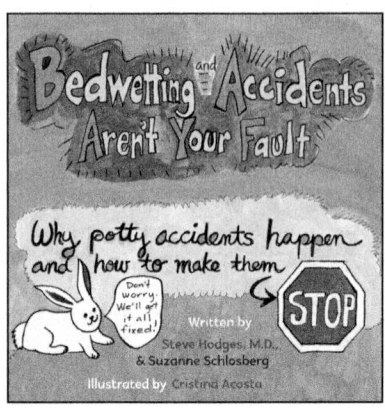

Bedwetting and Accidents Aren't Your Fault

"Terrific! The illustrations are so much fun they remove any possible embarrassment."
– Laura Markham, Ph.D., author of Peaceful Parent, Happy Kids: How to Stop Yelling and Start Connecting

"Dr. Pooper is a ROCKSTAR!!! I'd remind my son, 'What does Dr. Pooper want you to do every day?' and that would convince him to give it a try!"
– verified amazon purchaser

"Every pediatrician should refer the book — it is that good."
– verified amazon purchaser

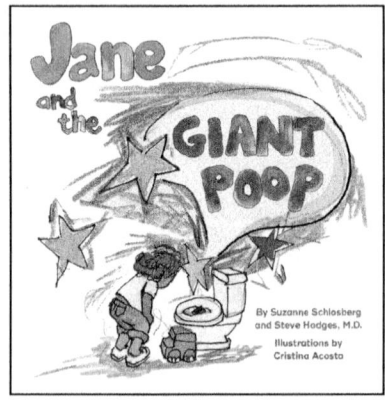

Jane and the Giant Poop

"Beautiful illustrations and a wonderful message about taking care of our bodies."
– Erin Wetjen, P.T., Pediatric Continence Specialist, Department of Urology, Mayo Clinic

"Very cute & engaging book. My kids read it 3 times first day it arrived. Helped 'normalize' their issue and bring humor to the process we are experiencing."
– verified amazon purchaser

"Not only captured my constipated 9-year old's attention, but all of his friends too! They were glued to the very end! "
– verified amazon purchaser

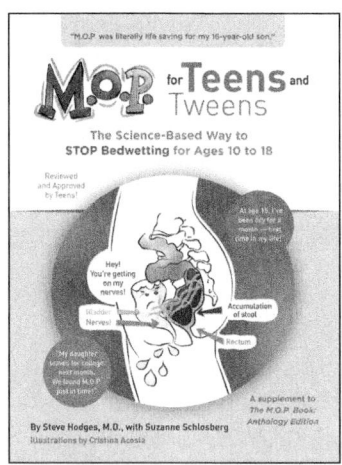

M.O.P. for Teens and Tweens

"This teen guide is a wonderful addition to the original M.O.P. book because my teen was able to personally read real-life experiences from other teens in the same boat."
– amazon reviewer

"This book explained everything without making me feel uncomfortable."
– 15-year-old with enuresis

"Thanks to this book, I know I'm not the only teenager dealing with bedwetting, and it is not my fault."
– 14-year-old with enuresis

"Your bedwetting teen NEEDS this book!"
– amazon reviewer

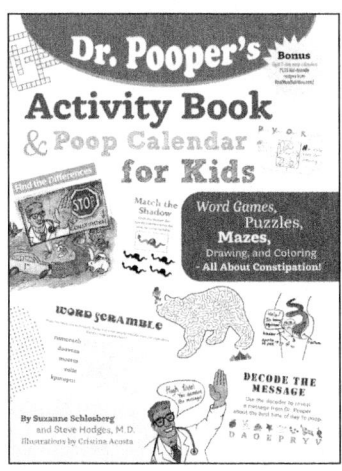

Dr. Pooper's Activity Book and Poop Calendar for Kids

"A great resource for kids with constipation and potty accidents! It helps them talk about it without embarrassment."
– Mike Garrett, M.D., Family Physician, Direct MD, Austin, TX

"My 5 y.o., who is following M.O.P., loves this activity book. He likes the mazes and 'spot the difference' pictures, and it's good for getting him talking about his potty issues."
– verified amazon purchaser

"Clever book! There is really a lot to do. I would never have thought constipation could be the subject of an activity book, but the authors did a really great job."
– verified amazon purchaser

Available in paperback on Amazon or in .pdf format at BedwettingAndAccidents.com.

143

Books and Guides for Parents and Health Professionals

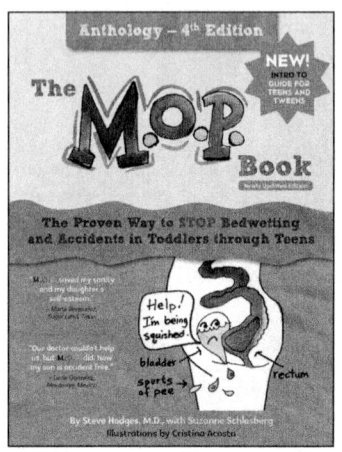

The M.O.P. Book: Anthology Edition

"M.O.P. saved my sanity and my daughter's self-esteem."
~ Marta Bermudez, Sugar Land, TX

"This book is a LIFESAVER!!! I cannot adequately express how it has helped my family."
~ verified amazon purchaser

"It is my mission to get the word out about how incredibly effective M.O.P. is."
~ Erin Wetjen, P.T., Specialist In Pediatric Incontinence Mayo Clinic, Rochester, MN

"I've learned more from this book than I have from countless doctor visits over the years."
~verified amazon purchaser

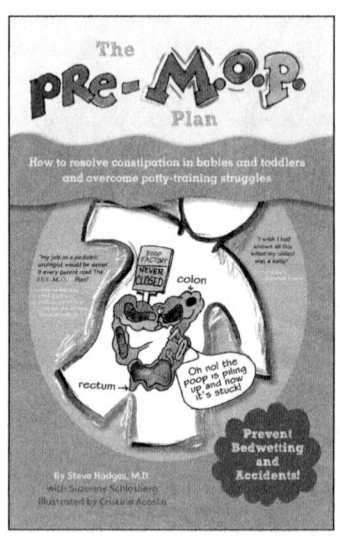

The Pre-M.O.P. Plan

"A book that will change lives! So many of the problems I treat could be prevented by Pre-M.O.P."
~ Irina Stanasel, M.D. Pediatric Urologist, UT Southwestern Medical Center, Dallas, Texas

"This book gave me the confidence to relieve my 2.5 year old's constipation. I went from feeling helpless, hopeless, and incredibly frustrated to feeling in control."
~ verified amazon purchaser

"Mandatory reading for all pediatric care providers!"
~ Rob Paynter, M.D., Pediatrician Novant Health Forsyth Pediatrics, Winston-Salem, North Carolina

"This creative book recognizes the important relationship between the colon and the urinary system."
~ Marc A. Levitt, M.D. Chief, Colorectal and Pelvic Reconstructive Surgery, Children's National Hospital Washington, D.C.

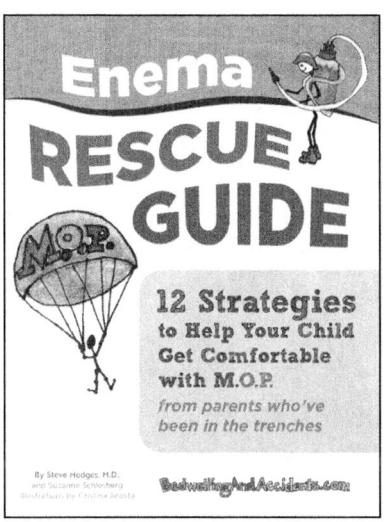
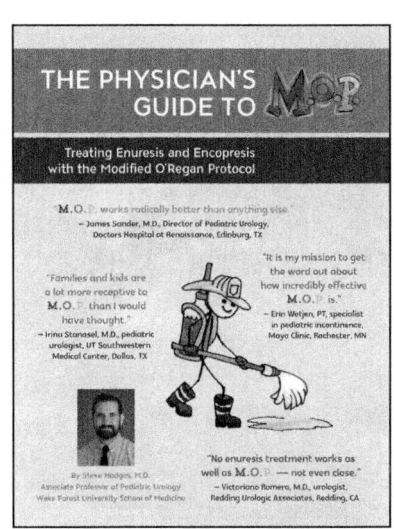
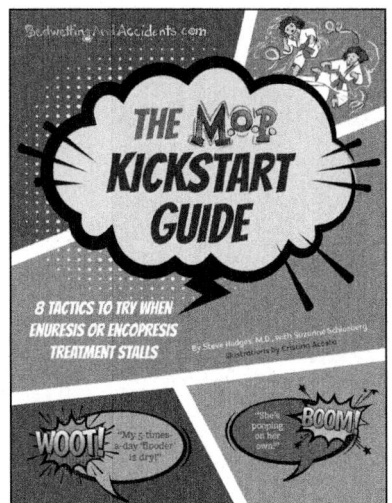
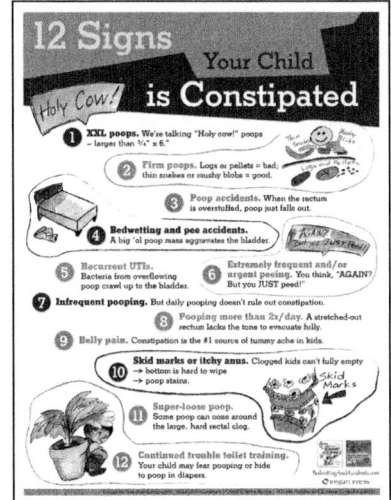

ABOUT THE AUTHORS AND THE ILLUSTRATOR

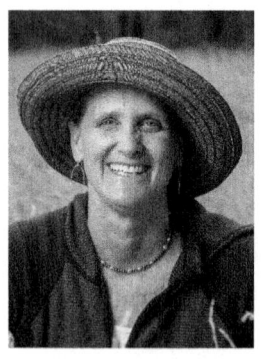

Suzanne Schlosberg is a health and parenting writer who specializes in translating clinical mumbo jumbo into stuff that's fun to read. Years ago, on a mission to achieve a diaper-free household in record time, Suzanne potty-trained her twin boys too early. She used Steve Hodges' methods to undo the damage and went on to found BedwettingAndAccidents.com with Dr. Hodges. The author or co-author of 20 books, Suzanne lives with her husband and teenage boys in Bend, Oregon. Her website is SuzanneSchlosbergWrites.com.

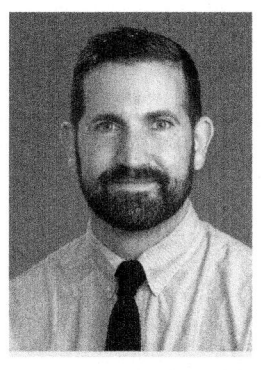

Steve Hodges is a professor of pediatric urology at Wake Forest University School of Medicine and an authority on childhood toileting issues. He has authored numerous journal articles and co-authored eight books with Suzanne Schlosberg. His mission is to dispel the myths, pervasive in popular culture and in medical literature, about enuresis and encopresis and to communicate to families that accidents are never a child's fault. Dr. Hodges lives in Winston-Salem, North Carolina, with his wife and three daughters. He blogs at BedwettingAndAccidents.com.

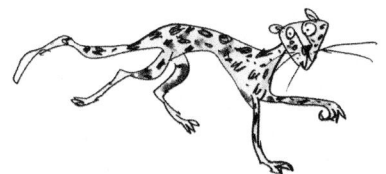

Mark Beech is a UK-based illustrator whose work is popular in the world of children's publishing. Mark has been illustrating professionally for over 20 years and has been scribbling since he was old enough to hold a pen. He has illustrated books for Sir Terry Pratchett, Jo Nesbø, Anthony Horowitz, and Enid Blyton, to name a few. Please take a look at more of Mark's work at MarkBeechIllustration.com.

NOTES

Here are a few facts to know about Emma and the E Club:

- The ancient Egyptians really did use enemas (p. 59), and Keeper of the Royal Rectum was an actual job, according to *A History of Medicine* by Lois N. Magner (CRC Press, 1992).

- Dr. Sean O'Regan (p. 94) is a retired doctor who did, in fact, practice in Canada in the 1980s and did pioneer the use of enemas for the treatment of enuresis. The story recounted in Chapter 18 is true and is described in greater detail in *The M.O.P. Book: Anthology Edition*, by Steve Hodges, M.D., with Suzanne Schlosberg (O'Regan Press, 2020).

- Charlotte's Bathtub Book Hook invention (p. 95) is based on a real 8-year-old's invention, described here: https://boingboing.net/2013/05/03/8-year-olds-invention-for-ke.html